C Bears

THE LONDON
PRINCESS ALEXANDR...
PROFESSIO...

NUMBER OF BOOK 17,720 CLASS 10A
This book may be taken out for a period not

exceeding 21 days.

Date	Date	Date
2 OCT 1981		
26 OCT 1981		
1 FEB 1982		

A Summary
of Medicine

A Summary of Medicine

For Nurses and Medical Auxiliaries

R. Gordon Cooke, M.D., M.R.C.S., L.R.C.P.

formerly Medical Superintendent, City Hospital, Derby, Examiner to the General Nursing Council for England and Wales.

Revised by Ann C. Miller, M.R.C.P.

FABER & FABER
3 Queen Square, London

*First published in 1945
by Faber & Faber Ltd
3 Queen Square London WC1
Second impression 1946
Second edition 1953
Third edition 1957
Reprinted 1958
Fourth edition 1963
Fifth edition 1966
Sixth edition 1973
Reprinted 1974
Seventh edition 1977
Printed in Great Britain
by Whitstable Litho Ltd., Whitstable
All rights reserved*

British Library Cataloguing in Publication Data

Cooke, Ralph Gordon
A summary of medicine for nurses and medical auxiliaries – 7th ed.
1. Pathology
I. Title II. Miller, Ann Christine
616'.002'4613   RB112
ISBN 0-571-04942-7

CONDITIONS OF SALE
*This book is sold subject to the condition that it shall not,
by way of trade or otherwise, be lent, re-sold, hired out
or otherwise circulated without the publisher's prior
consent in any form of binding or cover other than that in
which it is published and without a similar condition
including this condition being imposed on the subsequent
purchaser*

© R. Gordon Cooke and Ann Christine Miller 1973 and 1977.

Preface to the First Edition

It is not intended that this book should be read as a textbook of medicine for nurses. It is only an outline, and is meant for use in revision and for reference. Explanations are omitted as these are available in standard textbooks. I am much indebted to Dr. A. P. M. Page and to the late Mr. C. W. Stewart of Messrs. Faber and Faber for many helpful suggestions.

1945 R.G.C.

Preface to the Sixth Edition

The revision for this edition was carried out by Dr. Ann Miller who will be responsible for future editions.

1972 R.G.C.

Preface to the Seventh Edition

This book has been revised to keep in line with the latest developments.

1976 A.C.M.

ADDISON'S DISEASE

Condition. Deficiency of adrenal cortical hormones.

Cause. Bilateral disease of the adrenal glands (e.g. atrophy, tuberculosis).

Symptoms and Signs. Weakness. Anorexia, nausea, vomiting. Pigmentation of skin. Low systolic blood pressure (80-90 mm Hg). Hypoglycaemia. Symptoms may be accentuated at any time causing a 'crisis'.

Treatment. Cortisone and fludrocortisone, especially in crisis. (With fludrocortisone salt replacement now usually unnecessary.)

Special Tests. Plasma cortisol low and does not rise after giving A.C.T.H. Urinary steroid excretion low. X-ray for calcification of adrenals. Blood sugar and electrolytes.

Other Points. A rare disease. Infections may precipitate a crisis. Other forms of tuberculosis (e.g. pulmonary) may be present. Removal of adrenals may produce similar symptoms unless treated as above.

AGRANULOCYTOSIS

Condition. Severe reduction of polymorph white blood cells.

Causes. May be unknown. May be secondary to certain drugs (e.g. sulphonamides, chloramphenicol, antithyroid drugs, phenylbutazone, gold injections) or as part of aplastic anaemia.

Symptoms and Signs. General weakness. Fever. Ulceration of mouth and throat. Very susceptible to infections, including septicaemia.

Treatment. Withdrawal of drug (if cause). Barrier nursing (to avoid infection). Antibiotics. Local treatment to mouth.

Special Tests. Regular blood count if condition likely to arise. Marrow biopsy.

Blood Picture. Polymorph white count extremely low.

Other Points. May be rapidly fatal. Mild type may occur. May be due to an idiosyncrasy. With ulcerated throat, called 'agranulocytic angina'. Patients who recover warned against repetition of drug, if cause.

ALCOHOLISM (CHRONIC)

Condition. Addiction and illness due to chronic excessive alcohol intake.

Symptoms and Signs. Vague indigestion and poor appetite. Smells of alcohol. Defective memory. Personal carelessness. Loss of sense of time and place. Tremor. Fits. Peripheral neuritis.

Complications. Delirium tremens: noisy and hallucinated (especially after injuries or operations or in acute disease, e.g. pneumonia). Pneumonia. Dementia. Vitamin B deficiency. Heart failure. Cirrhosis of liver (can cause haematemesis).

Treatment. Careful nursing. Withdrawal of alcohol (may be gradual). Sedatives. 'Antabuse'. Vitamins, especially B vitamins. Symptomatic treatment.

Other Points. Co-operation of relatives important. May require removal to mental hospital or special institution. 'Alcoholics Anonymous' Association may help.

ALLERGY

Condition. Abnormal sensitivity reaction to substance foreign to body.

Causes. Substance may be (a) inhaled, e.g. pollens, (b) ingested, e.g. fish or drugs, (c) injected, e.g. serum sickness, or (d) in contact with skin, e.g. metals, detergents.

Symptoms and Signs. Various Forms: anaphylactic shock: serum sickness (which presents 6 to 12 days after injection—accompanied by urticaria, lymphadenopathy, arthralgia, oedema, fever): rhinitis (hay fever): asthma (which, however, is not always allergic in origin): skin reactions (urticaria, angioneurotic oedema, eczema, etc.): abdominal symptoms (pain, diarrhoea).

Treatment. Adrenaline. Antihistamines. Sometimes desensitization. Occasionally steroids. Avoid reactions to drugs or serum by asking patient about allergies, and giving test dose.

Special Test. Skin tests for sensitivity.

Other Points. This is one way in which the immunological mechanism, which protects the body against bacteria and foreign materials, may go wrong. Others are (1) allergic reactions to bacteria (acute glomerulonephritis, rheumatic fever); (2) reactions to body's own tissues (connective tissue disorders, Hashimoto's thyroiditis).

ANAEMIA (APLASTIC)

Condition. A severe anaemia arising from the failure of red cell formation in the bone marrow.

Causes. Usually unknown. Sometimes secondary to certain drugs (e.g. anticonvulsants, chloramphenicol, nitrogen mustards and other cytotoxic drugs) or exposure to X-rays, radium, etc. May be terminal state of other types of anaemia.

Occurrence. Those with unknown cause usually young adults. Others may be any age.

Symptoms and Signs. Weakness. Pallor. Dyspnoea. Haemorrhage into skin and from mucous membranes.

Treatment. Remove cause if known. Repeated transfusions. Try Steroids. Avoid or treat infections.

Special Tests. Blood count. Marrow biopsy. Bleeding time increased.

Blood Picture. Haemoglobin and red cell count very low. Cells have normal appearance. No reticulocytes. White cell and platelet counts low.

Other Points. May be rapidly fatal, or persist for months or even years, or occasionally recover.

ANAEMIA (HAEMOLYTIC)

Condition. Anaemia due to excessive destruction of red cells. Acute or chronic.

Causes.

(1) Fragile red cells (hereditary spherocytosis, sickle cell anaemia, etc.).

(2) Haemolytic substances—poisons (sulphonamides, lead, arsenic, snake venom), infections (malaria, septicaemia), antibodies (haemolytic disease of newborn, idiopathic acquired haemolytic anaemia, incompatible blood transfusion), leukaemia and other malignancies, burns, etc.

Symptoms and Signs. Acute—weakness, pyrexia, perhaps shock and anuria, symptoms of 'crisis'.

Chronic—anaemia, weakness, slight jaundice. Spleen and liver often enlarged. May develop pigment gall-stones.

Special Tests. Haemoglobin and red cell count diminished, but increased rate of red cell formation (reticulocytes in blood). Red cells normal colour; may be of abnormal shape and fragile in type (1). Serum bilirubin raised. Urinary urobilinogen increased but bilirubin rarely found. Faecal urobilinogen increased. Coombs' test positive if antibodies present.

Treatment. Some familial (type 1) cases require no treatment. Transfusion may be needed in 'crisis'. Splenectomy in hereditary spherocytosis ('acholuric family jaundice'). Treat cause if due to infection or poison. Idiopathic acquired haemolytic anaemia—A.C.T.H. or steroids: splenectomy sometimes beneficial. Exchange transfusion for haemolytic disease of newborn.

Other Points. In type (1), 'haemolytic crises' may occur, with increase in anaemia and jaundice, also fever, malaise and sometimes vomiting and abdominal pain. In sickle cell anaemia, crises may be precipitated by hypoxia, e.g. anaesthetics.

ANAEMIA (IRON DEFICIENCY)
(Also called 'microcytic' or 'hypochromic' anaemia.)

Condition. Anaemia due to iron deficiency.

Causes. Blood loss (menstruation, peptic ulcer, piles, etc.). Deficient diet. Malabsorption. Increased needs in pregnancy.

Occurrence. Commonest in women of child-bearing age.

Symptoms and Signs. Weakness. Easily tired and breathless. Indigestion. Pallor. Smooth tongue. Spoon-shaped nails (koilonychia).

Complication. Plummer-Vinson syndrome—sore tongue and difficulty in swallowing due to oesophageal web, with predisposition to pharyngeal carcinoma.

Treatment. Treat cause. Good food. Diet rich in iron (meat, eggs, green vegetables, lentils, peas, oatmeal). Iron, oral or parenteral. Attend to any source of blood loss. Transfusion occasionally required. For Plummer-Vinson syndrome, also vitamin B and if necessary pass bougies.

Special Tests. Blood count. Measurement of red cell parameters. Serum iron and iron binding capacity.

Blood Picture. Haemoglobin, red cell count and cell size all diminished. Reticulocyte count increased.

ANAEMIA (PERNICIOUS)

Cause. Absence of the 'intrinsic' factor in gastric secretion which is needed for absorption of vitamin B_{12}.

Occurrence. Most common in middle age.

Symptoms and Signs. Weakness. Pallor. Yellowish skin. Dyspnoea on slight exertion. Sore tongue. Indigestion. Tingling and numbness in fingers and toes. Unsteady gait.

Complications. Subacute combined degeneration of spinal cord (anaesthesia and paralysis of legs). Liability to sepsis. Increased risk of gastric carcinoma.

Treatment. Vitamin B_{12} by injection. Iron if coexistent iron deficiency. Transfusions occasionally. If cord damage present, physiotherapy.

May Resemble. Other types of megaloblastic anaemia due to deficiency of vitamin B_{12} (but with normal gastric secretion) or of folic acid.

Special Tests. Blood count. Marrow biopsy. Augmented histamine test (achlorhydria always present).

Blood Picture. Red cell count very low. Haemoglobin low. Large red cells (macrocytes) in blood, megaloblasts in marrow. Rising reticulocyte count indicates response to treatment.

Other Points. Vitamin B_{12} therapy, controlled by periodic blood counts, must be given for rest of life. If untreated, fatal in two or three years. If treated satisfactorily has normal life expectancy. Liver extracts not now used. Also called Addison's anaemia.

ANAEMIA (SICKLE CELL)

Condition. Severe anaemia due to abnormality of haemoglobin in red blood cells, leading to presence of sickle-shaped cells in bloodstream.

Cause. Inherited disease.

Occurrence. Two types: sickle cell anaemia (homozygote), sickle trait (heterozygote). Those with sickle trait only are usually asymptomatic. Occurs usually in negroes in tropical Africa and North America.

Symptoms and Signs. Severe form presents in childhood with anaemia, heart failure, jaundice, splenomegaly, thrombotic episodes and chronic ulceration of the legs. Splenic infarcts common in thrombotic episodes (crises).

Treatment. No treatment is curative, but blood transfusion, oxygen therapy may be helpful. Death is inevitable, usually before the age of thirty. Splenectomy is not usually helpful.

Blood Picture. Severe anaemia. Sickle test is positive. Haemoglobin electrophoresis distinguishes between the homozygous and the milder heterozygous form.

Other Points. Patients should avoid anoxia, e.g. unpressurized aircraft. Anaesthetists should maintain good oxygenation of those with sickle trait.

ANEURYSM (THORACIC)

Condition. An abnormal protrusion or swelling of the thoracic aorta.

Causes. Syphilis. Atheroma. Trauma (war wounds).

Occurrence. Usually in middle life. Much commoner in men.

Symptoms and Signs. Pain in chest and back. Unequal pulses. Those of Mediastinal Obstruction, see p. 81.

Treatment. Rest. Avoid constipation and excitement. Penicillin and potassium iodide, if syphilitic. Surgical treatment.

May Resemble. Aortic valve disease. Carcinoma of lung. Tumours of mediastinal glands. Dissecting aneurysm resembles myocardial infarction or pulmonary embolism or occasionally acute abdomen (*see* Cholecystitis, p. 28.)

Special Tests. X-ray. Serological tests for syphilis.

Other Points. Varieties. Saccular: local swelling of aorta. *Fusiform:* general dilatation. *Dissecting:* blood infiltrates between arterial wall layers.

May last a few years or sudden death may occur at any time. Death usually due to rupture, heart failure, or pulmonary complications. Dissecting aneurysm is itself very frequently fatal. Rarer now than formerly owing to extensive treatment of syphilis. Abdominal aortic aneurysm, due to atheroma, becoming commoner.

ANKYLOSING SPONDYLITIS

Condition. Arthritis of spine, leading to immobility (ankylosis).

Cause. Unknown.

Occurrence. Usually young men.

Symptoms and Signs. Insidiously progressive pain and stiffness of spine (starts like 'lumbago'). Severe kyphosis with poor chest expansion is common eventually.

Complications. Other joints may become involved. Iritis. Aortic incompetence.

May Resemble. Rheumatoid or osteo-arthritis of spine.

Treatment. Sleep on fracture boards, with pillow under back but not under head. Postural exercises. Analgesics. Phenylbutazone. Occasionally steroids. Radiotherapy. Rarely orthopaedic surgery.

Special Test. X-ray spine ('bamboo spine').

Other Points. May occur in psoriasis, ulcerative colitis, Crohn's disease.

ANOREXIA NERVOSA

Condition. Severe loss of appetite of psychological cause.

Cause. Emotional disturbance—usually anxiety, with hysterical or obsessional origin.

Occurrence. Usually young, unmarried women.

Symptoms and Signs. Prolonged aversion to food. Weight loss, amenorrhoea, downy body hair.

May Resemble. Hypopituitarism.

Treatment. Psychotherapy, usually in hospital. Persuasion to eat small tempting meals.

ANTIBIOTICS

Nature. Antibacterial substances derived from living organisms, usually moulds (or synthetic substances resembling them).

Uses. Ideally, the organism causing the disease—pneumonia, meningitis, pyelonephritis, septicaemia, etc.—should be isolated in the laboratory from the sputum, cerebro-spinal fluid, urine or blood. The pathologist then determines to which antibiotic the organism is sensitive. Empirical treatment may be needed until the results of laboratory tests are available.

INDIVIDUAL ANTIBIOTICS

CHLORAMPHENICOL

Administration. Drops, solution, cream. Oral or injection.

Uses. 'Broad spectrum antibiotic' (i.e. attacks wide range of organisms), used topically in eye, ear, but systemic use reserved for life-threatening infection such as typhoid, typhus, H. influenzae because of risk of aplastic anaemia.

Side Effects. Stomatitis, nausea, vomiting, diarrhoea. High doses in premature babies may lead to circulatory collapse.

Special Tests. Frequent blood counts (white cells and reticulocytes) to watch for marrow depression.

PENICILLIN

Administration. By intramuscular injection (when may be combined with procaine in slowly absorbed form), by tablets or in liquid form.

Uses. Mainly effective against Gram-positive organisms—staphylococci, pneumococci, streptococci, tetanus, diphtheria, gonorrhoea, syphilis.

Side Effects. Some patients are sensitive and produce allergic reactions—urticaria, erythema, asthma, painful swollen joints, purpura, fever.

Other Points. Organisms (especially staphylococci) may become resistant to penicillin, and then other antibiotics must be used. Still the cheapest and least toxic antibiotic. New synthetic penicillins being produced, some of which have broader spectrum, e.g. ampicillin ('Penbritin').

STREPTOMYCIN

Administration. By injection for general action. Orally for intestinal action.

Uses. Effective against many Gram-negative organisms, e.g. E. coli, proteus. Used especially for tuberculosis, bacillary dysentery, and with penicillin in mixed infections.

Side Effects. Deafness and vertigo (permanent). Fever. Rash.

Other Points. Used alone it tends to produce resistant strains. Main use is in tuberculosis, combined with P.A.S. and isoniazid.

TETRACYCLINES

Administration. By mouth or by injection.

Activity. 'Broad-spectrum antibiotic'. Highly effective against wide variety of bacteria and against rickettsia, spirochaetes and some large viruses.

Uses. Chest infections. Infections not responding to penicillin or sulphonamides. Rickettsial infections. Brucellosis. Whooping cough.

Side Effects. Stomatitis, nausea, vomiting and diarrhoea. Bowel may be invaded by resistant organisms, e.g. staphylococci or fungi. Skin rashes common.

Other Points. Group includes tetracycline, oxytetracycline, chlortetracycline, methacycline. May be used in penicillin-sensitive patients or penicillin-resistant infections.

OTHER ANTIBIOTICS

Synthetic penicillins—cloxacillin, methicillin, ampicillin. Erythromycin and cephaloridine (penicillin-resistant organisms). Neomycin (intestinal bactericide). Colistin ('Colomycin'), carbenicillin ('Pyopen') (Pseudomonas pyocyanea). Nystatin (yeast infections, e.g. thrush). Nitrofurantoin ('Furadantin') and nalidixic acid ('Negram') (urinary infections). Gentamicin ('Genticin'), fusidic acid ('Fucidin') for penicillin-resistant staphylococci.

New antibiotics are being constantly introduced.

AORTIC VALVE DISEASE

Condition. Deformity of aortic valve of heart. *Stenosis*—narrowing of orifice. *Incompetence*—failure to close in diastole, causing regurgitation of blood from aorta into left ventricle.

Causes. Usually rheumatic endocarditis. Stenosis may be congenital (or perhaps arteriosclerotic in old age). Incompetence may be due to syphilis, aneurysm, bacterial endocarditis.

Occurrence. Commoner in men.

Symptoms and Signs. Breathlessness, fainting and angina, especially in stenosis. Heart failure in both. Pulse—plateau type (slow rise and fall) in stenosis; collapsing or 'water hammer' in incompetence. Pulse pressure—difference between systolic and diastolic blood pressure, low in stenosis, high in incompetence. Large heart. Murmurs—systolic in stenosis, diastolic in incompetence.

Complications. Heart block and Stokes-Adams attacks, especially in stenosis. Bacterial endocarditis may cause further damage to an already abnormal valve.

Treatment. Limit activity. Surgical treatment is improving (by dilating or replacing valves). Treat heart failure or complications.

Special Tests. Chest X-ray. E.C.G. Blood tests for syphilis. Blood cultures if bacterial endocarditis suspected.

ARTERIAL DEGENERATION

(ARTERIOSCLEROSIS AND ATHEROMA)

Condition. Degeneration of arterial walls, with formation of thrombus and plaques which may occlude lumen.

Causes. Unknown. Always occurs to some extent in old age. Accelerated by diabetes mellitus. Probably accelerated by inactivity, obesity, dietary factors (e.g. animal fat), high blood cholesterol, smoking, hypertension, psychological stress.

Occurrence. Commoner in males.

Symptoms and Signs. Hardened, tortuous arteries may be felt in various sites and seen in optic fundi. May restrict blood supply to various organs, or artery wall may give way and produce haemorrhage. May thus cause cerebrovascular accident and cerebral ischaemia, ischaemic heart disease, gangrene, intermittent claudication, hypertension and other disorders.

Treatment. Unsatisfactory. The following may sometimes be helpful. Avoid smoking. *Diet:* prevent obesity and perhaps avoid animal fats. *Surgery:* arterial reconstruction if practicable; sympathectomy (helps skin circulation only). *Drugs:* control hypertension; vasodilators in ischaemic heart disease; occasionally anticoagulants; perhaps reduce blood cholesterol.

ASTHMA (BRONCHIAL)

Condition. Periodic paroxysmal attacks of wheezing and dyspnoea. Spasm of the bronchioles occurs, causing difficulty in expiration.

Causes. Allergic: emanations from animals, pollen of grasses, certain foods. Infective: sinusitis, bronchitis. Psychological. Often no apparent cause.

Occurrence. Usually starts in early life. Common in overanxious, intelligent type. Relatives often have eczema, asthma or allergies.

Symptoms and Signs. Often rapid onset. Short inspirations with violent attempts at expiration. 'Tightness' and wheezing of chest. Rhonchi on auscultation. Cyanosis if very severe. Sputum when attack passes off. Anxiety. Attack may last minutes or hours, or persist as 'status asthmaticus'.

Complications. Emphysema. Cor pulmonale.

Treatment. In Attack. Reassurance. Isoprenaline inhaler. Ephedrine. Adrenaline subcutaneously. Aminophylline. Corticosteroids. Remove any allergic source. Avoid deep sleep, which depresses breathing efforts. Antibiotics if infection. *To avoid attacks.* Bronchodilators such as ephedrine, isoprenaline, orciprenaline, salbutamol. Treat respiratory infection promptly. Di-sodium cromoglycate ('Intal') is useful prophylactic. Skin tests for sensitivity to certain proteins and desensitization if practicable. Relaxation and breathing exercises. Phenobarbitone if of nervous origin. Severe cases may need long-term corticosteroids.

Special Tests. Skin tests as above. Sputum culture.

Nursing Points. Usually more comfortable sitting up, with plenty of fresh air. Oxygen in status asthmaticus.

Other Points. May pass off after some years (e.g. after puberty), or recur throughout life. Often occurs with chronic bronchitis. Similar attacks occur in 'cardiac asthma'—congestion of lungs due to heart disease.

ATRIAL FIBRILLATION

Condition. Disordered action of atria of heart, leading to irregular ventricular contractions.

Causes. Ischaemic heart disease. Rheumatic heart disease, particularly mitral stenosis. Thyrotoxicosis. Any myocardial degeneration.

Symptoms and Signs. Rapid pulse (up to 180), with total irregularity of rhythm and volume. Often different rates at apex and at wrist.

Complications. Heart failure. Especially with mitral stenosis, embolism from thrombi arising from heart (to brain, limbs, gut, etc.).

Treatment. Rest. Digitalis. Conversion to normal rhythm can be attempted (electrically or with quinidine), but carries risk of cerebral embolism if fibrillation long established. Treat thyrotoxicosis if cause.

Special Test. E.C.G.

Nursing Points. Watch for signs of digitalis poisoning. Record apex beat as well as pulse rate.

Other Point. May be paroxysmal at first, become permanent later.

BRONCHIECTASIS

Condition. Chronic dilatation of the terminal bronchioles associated with the production of much foul sputum.

Causes. Bronchopneumonia, bronchitis and whooping cough, especially in children. Cystic fibrosis. Tuberculosis. Obstruction of bronchi by inhaled foreign body or by lymph nodes enlarged by tuberculosis or tumour. Rarely congenital.

Symptoms and Signs. Large amount of foul sputum especially in morning. Paroxysmal cough. Offensive breath. Occasional haemoptysis. Febrile episodes. Clubbing of fingers. General signs and symptoms of chronic sepsis.

Complications. Bronchopneumonia. Empyema. Abscess of brain. Amyloid disease.

Treatment. Mild dry climate or locality with little or no atmospheric pollution if possible. Postural drainage. Breathing exercises. Antibiotics. Surgery (lobectomy) in some cases. Remove foreign body if present.

May Resemble. Chronic bronchitis. Abscess of lung. Pulmonary tuberculosis.

Special Tests. Chest X-ray. Bronchography (X-ray following injection of iodized oil down trachea). Sputum culture.

Nursing Points. Teach general hygiene and cleanliness. Avoid close proximity to other patients. Watch for undue discomfort during postural drainage.

BRONCHITIS (ACUTE)

Condition. Acute catarrhal inflammation of the bronchi.

Causes. Downward spread of infection, e.g. a 'cold'. Inhalation of irritants.

Occurrence. All ages. *Children:* common as complication of acute fevers including colds, and in under-nutrition. *Old Age:* common, especially in debility.

Symptoms and Signs. Those of a chest-cold. Cough, pain in chest—later fairly profuse sputum. May be wheezing and dyspnoea. Fever. Widespread signs on auscultation.

Complications. Bronchopneumonia. Acute cardiac failure in aged or those with lung or heart disease.

Treatment. Warmth. Hot drinks. Stop smoking. Inhalations if much spasm. Antibiotics. If cough dry and distressing, suppress with codeine linctus.

May Resemble. Pneumonia.

Special Tests. Sputum culture. Chest X-ray.

Nursing Points. Warm room. Prop patient up. Encourage expectoration. Bed jacket.

Other Points. Common in winter. Tendency to recur with development of chronic bronchitis.

BRONCHITIS (CHRONIC)

Condition. Chronic catarrhal inflammation of the bronchi and bronchioles. Liable to acute exacerbations.

Causes. Chronic irritation, e.g. by tobacco smoke or fumes, or recurrent infection.

Occurrence. Middle and old age. Commoner in males. Commoner in towns and among smokers. Worse in winter.

Symptoms and Signs. Morning cough with sputum. Dyspnoea. Rhonchi. Those of acute bronchitis in acute exacerbation.

Complications. Bronchopneumonia. Emphysema. Heart failure. Bronchiectasis. Respiratory failure.

Treatment. Mild and dry climate or locality with little or no atmospheric pollution, if practicable. Stop smoking. Bronchodilator drugs and possibly long-term antibiotic therapy. Breathing exercises. For exacerbation: as in Acute Bronchitis. Treat cardiac failure if impending. Treat respiratory failure (rising carbon dioxide in blood) with controlled oxygen—usually 28 per cent, as provided by a Ventimask as 100 per cent oxygen may cause respiratory arrest in this situation, respiratory stimulants, e.g. nikethamide or perhaps on respirator.

May Resemble. Bronchiectasis. Pulmonary tuberculosis. Carcinoma of bronchus.

Special Tests. Sputum culture. Chest X-ray. Respiratory function tests.

Other Points. Special care during winter. Treat exacerbation promptly. Tends to progress gradually, despite treatment, and to develop complications.

BRUCELLOSIS (UNDULANT FEVER)

Condition. Blood stream infection causing acute or chronic symptoms.

Cause. Brucella organism, strains of which may be found in cow's or goat's milk or in pigs.

Incubation Period. One to three weeks.

Symptoms and Signs. Weakness. Profuse sweating. Anorexia. Headaches. Pains in muscles and in back. Depression. Cough. Enlarged spleen. Fever, usually diurnal and brief but may be prolonged and undulate from day to day.

Treatment. Rest. Tetracycline. If chronic case—tetracycline and streptomycin, possibly for many weeks.

May Resemble. Tuberculosis. Subacute bacterial endo-carditis. Glandular fever. Typhoid fever. Malaria. Neurosis.

Special Tests. Blood culture. Agglutination reaction of blood.

Other Points. One of the causes of P.U.O. (pyrexia of unknown origin). Tetracycline usually effective. If untreated may run acute self-limiting or chronic relapsing courses. Common in Malta where goat's milk is much used ('Malta Fever'): otherwise usually due to cow's milk ('Abortus Fever'). Prevent Brucellosis by pasteurization of milk.

CEREBROVASCULAR ACCIDENT

Condition. Sudden interference with blood supply to the brain, by haemorrhage, thrombosis or embolism of cerebral artery.

Causes. Haemorrhage: arterial degeneration, especially with hypertension. *Thrombosis:* arterial degeneration, especially with hypotensive episode. *Embolism:* embolus from atrium in fibrillation, ventricle in myocardial infarction, or valve in bacterial endocarditis.

Occurrence. Mainly beyond middle age, especially males.

Symptoms and Signs. Variable: contralateral hemiplegia with upgoing plantar response commonest: perhaps aphasia, visual or sensory loss, convulsions, fever, stiff neck, papilloedema. Sudden onset, usually with coma, in haemorrhage and embolism. Progressive over hours or days in thrombosis. Patient may die (often of pneumonia in coma), or recover partially or completely. If power, etc. returns, it starts within a month but may improve for a year. Mental impairment and emotional lability often persist.

May Resemble. Other causes of coma.

Special Tests. Lumbar puncture (pressure and protein may be raised, with blood especially in haemorrhage).

Treatment. Rest. Warmth. As for coma if present. (Anticoagulants if diagnosis of thrombo-embolism is certain). Passive progressing to active movements. Occasionally, splinting to prevent deformity. Walking exercises and general rehabilitation.

Nursing Point. If loss of speech, tact in interpreting patient's wants.

Other Points. Cerebral arterial degeneration, without acute episodes, may produce dizziness on standing up, mental deterioration and epilepsy. Narrowing of carotid artery may give transient paralysis or blindness: demonstrated by arteriogram and sometimes treated by surgery or anticoagulants.

CHICKENPOX (VARICELLA)

Condition. An infectious disease characterized by slight malaise quickly followed by a vesicular rash.

Cause. The same virus as responsible for herpes zoster.

Occurrence. Very common. Very infectious. Chiefly children under ten.

Incubation Period. About 14 days.

Symptoms and Signs. Slight malaise (may be absent). Rash (1st or 2nd day), papules which rapidly become vesicles then pustules, widespread chiefly on trunk and face and in axilla—in contrast to smallpox. Spots occur in 'crops'.

Treatment. Bed for a period. Keep skin clean and dust with talcum powder: local antiseptics if infected. Antihistamines to relieve itching.

May Resemble. Smallpox. Herpes. Scabies. Papular urticaria.

Nursing Points. Isolation. Keep mouth clean, especially if vesicles inside. Cut hair if vesicles on scalp. Child's hands in gloves if tendency to scratch. Do not pick off crusts.

Other Points. Infectious until last crust has separated. Spontaneous recovery usual. May be an earlier rash of scarlatiniform type. May arise following contact with a case of herpes zoster.

CHOLECYSTITIS (ACUTE)

Condition. Inflammation of the gall bladder.

Cause. Obstruction to outflow of bile (usually by gall stone) with secondary infection.

Occurrence. Commonest in middle age and in females.

Symptoms and Signs. Epigastric pain, sometimes referred to right shoulder. Tenderness under right ribs. Flatulence, nausea, vomiting. Raised temperature and pulse. Occasionally jaundice.

Complications. Empyema or rupture of gall bladder. Chronic cholecystitis.

Treatment. Rest. Warm applications to abdomen. Analgesics for pain. Antibiotics.

May Resemble. Other causes of abdominal pain—appendicitis, perforated peptic ulcer, pancreatitis, intestinal obstruction, renal colic or urinary infection, ruptured ectopic pregnancy and gynaecological causes, aortic aneurysm, pleurisy, myocardial infarction. Also infective hepatitis.

Special Tests. Blood white cell count. Bilirubin in serum and urine. X-ray abdomen. Cholecystogram a few weeks after attack.

Other Points. Treatment of the condition is with antibiotics, but the diseased gall bladder is usually removed surgically as recurrences are common.

CHOREA (SYDENHAM'S)

Condition. A disease characterized by irregular spasmodic involuntary movements.

Cause. Probably related to rheumatic fever. May be precipitated by emotional upsets or mental strain, or by pregnancy ('chorea gravidarum').

Occurrence. Chiefly in children, especially girls. Also in pregnancy, especially first.

Symptoms and Signs. Quick, irregular, purposeless movements chiefly of hands and face. Movements cease during sleep. Emotionalism and irritability. Poor muscle tone.

Complication. Rheumatic carditis.

Treatment. Rest. Aspirin or other salicylates. Sedatives if necessary.

Nursing Points. Quietness—corner of ward. Prevent injury from restlessness. Help in feeding. Care of mouth. Take temperature in axilla.

Other Points. Usually lasts some weeks. Tends to recur. Also called 'St Vitus' Dance'.

CHOREA (HUNTINGTON'S)

Condition. Hereditary disease, presenting usually in middle life with chorea (faster and more jerky than in Sydenham's) and later progressing to dementia. It is rare.

CIRRHOSIS OF LIVER

Condition. An increase in the fibrous tissue in the liver accompanied by necrosis and regeneration of liver cells.

Causes. Often unknown. Alcoholism. Dietary deficiencies, mainly protein. Chronic hepatitis or cholangitis due to infection or bile duct obstruction. Rarely chronic heart failure.

Occurrence. Middle age, especially males.

Symptoms and Signs. Liver may be enlarged or shrunken. Symptoms of portal hypertension: indigestion, enlarged spleen, haematemesis from oesophageal varices, haemorrhoids, enlarged veins on abdomen, anaemia, ascites. Symptoms of hepatic failure: may be jaundice, oedema, tendency to bleed, flapping tremor, foetor, spider naevi, red palms, confusion and coma in late stages.

Treatment. Regular life and habits. Exclude alcohol. High calorie diet rich in protein. Vitamins. But if mental confusion or coma, give glucose, neomycin and low protein. Haematemesis—transfusion, and vasopressin or inflatable Sengstaken tube if severe. Ascites—restrict fluids and salt, diuretics, paracentesis if causing discomfort. Surgical treatment for portal hypertension, e.g. portacaval anastomosis.

Special tests. Plasma proteins altered. Liver function tests abnormal. Prothrombin time increased.

Prognosis. Despite treatment, gradual worsening is usual. Hepatic failure and bleeding from oesophageal varices are often fatal.

COELIAC DISEASE

Condition. A type of intestinal malabsorption in children.

Cause. Hypersensitivity to gluten (protein in wheat and rye), producing abnormal gut mucosa.

Occurrence. Usually noticed on weaning.

Symptoms and Signs. Loss of appetite. Anaemia. Wasting with abdominal distension. Stunted growth. Diarrhoea with pale, bulky stools. If untreated, symptoms usually improve before puberty, but may persist into adult life.

Complications. Interference with calcium metabolism may cause rickets and tetany. Oedema. Scurvy. Liable to respiratory infections.

Treatment. Gluten-free diet for rest of life. At first, supplements of vitamins, iron, folic acid, calcium. Steroids in emergency.

May Resemble. Fibrocystic disease of pancreas ('mucoviscidosis'). Malnutrition. Congenital intestinal abnormalities.

Special Tests. Blood count. Serum iron, calcium, proteins, etc. Faecal fat content. Glucose or xylose tolerance test. Barium meal. Small intestinal biopsy.

Prognosis. With treatment, excellent.

COMA

Condition. Deep unconsciousness.

Causes.

1. *Cardio-vascular.* Stokes-Adams syndrome. Fainting attacks.
2. *Central Nervous System.* Cerebro-vascular accident, subarachnoid or other intra-cranial haemorrhage. Encephalitis or meningitis. Cerebral tumour or abscess. Epilepsy. Hypertensive encephalopathy. Eclampsia.
3. *Accident.* Head injury. Electric shock.
4. *Metabolic.* Diabetic ketosis, or hypoglycaemia (from insulin). Hypothermia, myxoedema or hypopituitarism, occasionally heat hyperpyrexia. Addisonian crisis. Uraemia. Hepatic failure.
5. *Poisoning.* Alcohol. Drugs (overdose of aspirin, barbiturates, etc.). Anaesthetics. Carbon monoxide or other poisoning.
6. *Psychiatric.* Catatonia. Hysteria. Coma may be simulated in malingering.
7. *Profound Hypotension.* Myocardial infarction, haemorrhage, anaphylactic shock, severe infections.
8. *Terminal State.* In various infections, malignant and other diseases.

Treatment. Treat cause if practicable, e.g. poisoning, surgical conditions. Maintain airway and fluid balance. Tube- or drip-feed. Catheterize bladder if necessary. Nurse on side, turning two-hourly. Watch for bed sores. Clean mouth. Avoid constipation. Passive movements.

CONGENITAL HEART DISEASE

Condition. An anatomical abnormality in the structure of the heart.

Cause. Congenital: may be failure of development or may be due to infectious disease while still *in utero*, especially Rubella (German measles).

Occurrence. From birth.

Symptoms and Signs. May be none if mild. Stunted growth, fatigue, dyspnoea, palpitations. If more severe, heart failure, fainting, angina, haemoptysis. In 'cyanotic' types, cyanosis and finger clubbing, and tendency to adopt squatting posture.

On auscultation: abnormal sounds with most types.

Complications. Bacterial endocarditis. Respiratory infections.

Treatment. Surgery if possible. Treat complications. Penicillin prior to dental procedures, to avoid bacterial endocarditis.

Prognosis. Varies with severity of lesion.

CONNECTIVE TISSUE DISORDERS
(COLLAGEN DISEASES)

Condition. A group of diseases involving widespread inflammation of connective tissue. Includes polyarteritis nodosum ('P.A.N.'), temporal arteritis, disseminated lupus erythematosus ('D.L.E.'), scleroderma (systemic sclerosis), dermatomyositis, polymyositis. Also possibly rheumatoid arthritis, rheumatic fever and glomerulonephritis.

Cause. Probably auto-immune reaction—sensitization to own bodily tissues.

Occurrence. Mostly in middle life. Temporal arteritis in older people.

Symptoms and Signs. Malaise. Recurrent fever. Weight loss. Anaemia (various types). Any system may be involved. Joint pain common in all (sometimes like rheumatoid arthritis). Renal damage (especially in P.A.N. and D.L.E.). Skin eruptions (especially D.L.E.). Hardening of skin and alimentary tract (especially scleroderma). Vomiting and diarrhoea, sometimes with blood (P.A.N.). Tender, weak muscles (dermatomyositis and polymyositis). Various lesions of lungs and pleura. Enlarged lymph nodes, liver and spleen. Arterial inflammation producing hypertension and infarction of various organs in P.A.N.; headaches and blindness in temporal arteritis. Myocardial degeneration, pericarditis (especially P.A.N. and D.L.E.). Polyneuritis. Sometimes mental changes (D.L.E.).

May Resemble. Many other diseases affecting the systems mentioned.

Special Tests. E.S.R. (high). Haemoglobin and blood film. L.E. cells in blood (especially D.L.E.). Biopsy muscle or skin (or temporal artery). X-ray joints and chest. Serum protein electrophoresis. Anti-nuclear factor (A.N.F.).

Treatment. May be necessary to give steroids, but are of variable value. Physiotherapy in arthritis or scleroderma.

Other Points. See also Rheumatoid Arthritis, Rheumatic Fever, and Allergy.

Prognosis. All except temporal arteritis tend to progress to ultimate death, polyarteritis being the most rapid (weeks or months) and scleroderma the least rapid (several years). Occasionally long remissions occur. Temporal arteritis subsides spontaneously, but may leave blindness (may be prevented by steroids).

CONVULSIONS (INFANTILE)

Condition. Loss of consciousness associated with convulsive movements.

Causes. Onset of febrile illness. Birth injury to brain, or asphyxia. Epilepsy. Cerebral diseases including meningitis. Tetany, uraemia or hypoglycaemia. Certain poisons.

Occurrence. Infancy.

Symptoms and Signs. May be only slight twitching, or child becomes unconscious with muscular rigidity and cyanosis followed by convulsive movements of limbs.

Treatment. Loosen collar, place on side, maintain airway. Tepid sponging if high fever. Sedatives. Anaesthesia, if severe. Treat primary cause.

Other Points. Children of an emotional type may hold their breath and become cyanosed and convulsed. See also Epilepsy.

Prognosis. Febrile—excellent. Others—according to cause.

CRANIAL NERVES (DISEASES OF)

Tumours, cerebral arterial disease (cerebrovascular accident or degeneration), meningitis, encephalitis, syphilis, trauma or skull fracture may cause lesions of any cranial nerves. For other causes see below.

1*st. Olfactory.* Results in loss of sense of smell and flavour.

Causes. Nasal inflammation (colds, smoking).

2*nd. Optic.* Results in defective vision or blindness.

Causes. Diabetes mellitus, hypertension, aneurysms, disseminated sclerosis. (Other conditions can cause defective vision, e.g. brain damage or tumour, thrombosis of central retinal artery or vein, glaucoma, cataract, corneal scars.)

3rd, 4th and 6th. Result in squint, double vision, ptosis, unequal or unreactive pupils.

Causes. Aneurysms, disseminated sclerosis, myasthenia gravis.

5th. *Trigeminal.* (a) Trigeminal neuralgia ('tic douloureux'): recurrent, very severe stabbing pains and numbness in face and head. *Cause* unknown; usually in old people. *Treat* with sedatives, alcohol injection into Gasserian ganglion, or division of nerve roots.

(b) Herpes zoster of ophthalmic division may cause corneal ulcer.

(c) In lesion of motor root, jaw deviates to affected side.

7th. *Facial.* Results in facial paralysis or spasm. Sometimes loss of taste on front of tongue and reduced salivation.

Causes. Infections of ear and nasopharynx. Tumour or injury (e.g. at operation) of parotid gland. 'Bell's Palsy'—inflammation of nerve, cause unknown.

8th. *Acoustic (cochlear and vestibular).* Results in deafness, tinnitus, vertigo, nystagmus.

Causes. Drugs (quinine, streptomycin, etc.), disseminated sclerosis. (Similar symptoms and signs may result from diseases of ear, e.g. otitis media, otosclerosis, or of labyrinth, e.g. Ménière's syndrome, vestibulitis.)

9th. *Glossopharyngeal.* Results in difficulty in swallowing (also, rarely, glossopharyngeal neuralgia).

10th. *Vagus.* Results in difficulty in swallowing, hoarseness, sometimes cough, tachycardia.

11th. *Accessory.* Results in weakness of neck movements and of shrugging shoulders.

12th. *Hypoglossal.* Results in weakness or deviation of tongue.

Causes of lesions of 9th, 10th, 11th and 12th. Lymph nodes in neck. Aortic aneurysm, tumours in chest or neck or operations on thyroid may cause hoarseness through damage to recurrent laryngeal branch of vagus. Cerebral haemorrhage and other brain lesions.

CRETINISM

Condition. Defective development due to absence or deficiency of thyroid gland.

Cause. Congenital.

Symptoms and Signs. Coarse features. Dry skin. Coarse hair. Large tongue. Mental dullness. Slow growth. Umbilical hernia. Low metabolic rate. Constipation.

Treatment. Thyroxine for rest of life.

May Resemble. Mongolism. Other causes of mental deficiency.

Other Points. Great improvement if treated very early. If untreated, progressive mental deterioration.

CUSHING'S SYNDROME

Condition. Excessive quantity of adrenocortical steroid hormones.

Causes.

1. Tumour or over-action of pituitary gland or adrenal cortex.
2. Treatment with corticosteroid drugs (cortisone, hydrocortisone, prednisolone, etc.) or A.C.T.H.

Symptoms and Signs. 'Moon-face' and 'buffalo hump' (soft tissue swelling over upper thoracic spine). Striae on abdomen. Bruising. Acne. Fluid retention (weight gain, oedema). Hypertension. Osteoporosis (back pain, fractured vertebrae). Peptic ulcer. Glycosuria or diabetes mellitus. Amenorrhoea, hirsutism. Liability to infection. Weakness. Emotional change, even psychosis.

Special tests. Urinary steroids estimation. Plasma cortisol (hydrocortisone). X-ray abdomen, bones and skull. Tests of pituitary function.

Treatment.
For (1). Often bilateral adrenalectomy (and replacement therapy as for Addison's disease).
For (2). Reduce dose as far as possible. Possibly calcium and anabolic drugs may delay osteoporosis. Treat individual features.

Other Points. Steroid therapy must never be stopped suddenly and dose must be increased if infection, accident, operation or other stress occurs. This is because patient's adrenal cortex will not function normally for up to two years after a long course of steroids.

CYSTIC DISEASE OF KIDNEYS

Condition. Defective development of kidneys which are much enlarged with numerous cysts.

Cause. Congenital.

Occurrence. Symptoms often unnoticed till middle age.

Symptoms and Signs. Bilateral renal tumour. Pain. Haematuria. Hypertension. Symptoms of chronic renal failure.

Complications. Uraemia. Cerebral haemorrhage. Congestive heart failure.

Treatment. Palliative. Symptomatic.

Special Tests. Plain X-ray and intravenous pyelogram. Blood urea (raised). Blood pressure (raised).

Other Points. Usually fatal in middle age, but mild cases may have no symptoms and be diagnosed at post-mortem. A rare disease. Also called 'polycystic disease of kidneys'.

CYSTIC FIBROSIS
(FIBROCYSTIC DISEASE OF THE PANCREAS)

Condition. Inherited disease in which mucus secretions are abnormally thick.

Cause. Recessively inherited. Abnormality of salt excretion.

Occurrence. Usually in infancy, but may survive to adult life.

Complications. Meconium ileus at birth, failure to thrive, recurrent chest infections and bronchiectasis, pancreatic insufficiency and intestinal malabsorption. Eventually cirrhosis of liver.

Treatment. Antibiotics and physiotherapy for chest infections. Saline nebulizer to reduce mucus stickiness. Pancreatic enzyme supplements.

Special tests. Sweat test, chest X-ray, tryptic activity of stool.

Other points. With intensive treatment patients may survive to adult life.

CYSTITIS

Condition. Inflammation of the bladder.

Causes. Ascending infection—from urethra. Descending infection—from kidney. Spread from adjacent pelvic infection.

Occurrence. At any age. Commoner in females.

Symptons and Signs. Frequency of micturition. Dysuria. Cloudy urine, perhaps haematuria. Pain in lower abdomen.

Treatment. Give fluids freely. Mixtures to make urine alkaline, e.g. potassium citrate. Sulphonamides or antibiotics. Treatment of underlying cause.

Special Tests. Microscopy and culture (with sensitivity tests) of urine, including exclusion of tuberculosis. Intravenous pyelogram. Cystoscopy.

Other Points. May accompany enlargement of prostate, vesical calculi, strictures, pregnancy. May follow catheterization, especially without proper asepsis. Often accompanied by pyelonephritis. May follow radiotherapy to the pelvis.

DEPRESSION

Condition. Depression of mood and mental activity.

Types.

1. (a) Psychoses especially manic-depressive.
   (b) Associated with schizophrenia.
   (c) Senile—with or without dementia (used to be called 'involutional melancholia').
2. An excessive (neurotic) reaction to adverse events (e.g. bereavement, financial disaster).
3. Sequela of certain diseases (especially virus infections such as influenza, infective hepatitis, infectious mononucleosis), drugs (reserpine, barbiturates, sulphonamides) or the puerperium.

Symptoms and Signs. May come 'out of the blue' (without obvious precipitating factor) in type 1, or as part of gross cyclical alternation of mood in manic-depressive psychosis. In types 2 and 3, precipitating factor usually obvious.

Unhappiness, unwarranted pessimism, lack of energy, inability to concentrate, disturbance of sleep (especially waking early), headache, constipation, suicidal inclinations. In severe cases (especially type 1), guilt-feelings, slowness of thought and speech ('retardation'), social withdrawal. Anxiety, agitation and delusions may also be present. All symptoms tend to be worse in morning, least in evening.

Treatment. If mild, support and perhaps psychotherapy until attack passes. If more severe: 1. Supervision to prevent suicide, often in psychiatric hospital. 2. Drugs—(a) amitriptyline ('Tryptizol'), imipramine ('Tofranil'), (b) phenelzine ('Nardil') or other mono-amine oxidase inhibitors, (c) symptomatic treatment with tranquillizers or night-sedation. 3. Electro-convulsive therapy (E.C.T.). Occupational therapy often helpful. Commonest fault is to tell depressed patient to 'pull himself together' or 'snap out of it'; this he cannot do.

Nursing Points. Supervision depends mainly on nurses. Build up friendly but firm relationship, constantly reassuring but not blaming.

Other Points. Recovery from one episode usually occurs even without, but more quickly with treatment, but there is a tendency to recurrence in type 1 and perhaps type 2, especially if previous history or family history of depression, or if no obvious precipitating factor, or if underlying personality poor. Type 1 (a) sometimes called 'endogenous', type 2 'exogenous' or 'reactive'. Patients on mono-amine oxidase inhibitors must not take cheese, Marmite or certain drugs (may produce serious rise in blood-pressure).

DIABETES MELLITUS

Condition. Abnormal metabolism of carbohydrates and also of fats, with high blood sugar and glycosuria.

Cause. Deficiency of insulin (internal secretion of pancreas), or presence of antagonists to insulin.

Occurrence. All ages. More serious in the young. Elderly diabetics often obese.

Symptoms and Signs. Thirst. Polyuria. Dehydration. Loss of weight. Weakness. Pruritus vulvae.

Complications. Septic conditions, e.g. boils, toe infections. Atheroma. Gangrene. Peripheral neuropathy. Retinopathy.

Cataract. Chronic nephritis. Obstetric complications (and heavy babies). Pulmonary tuberculosis.

Hyperglycaemia and ketosis (in untreated diabetes, or from insufficient insulin) develops over hours or days, with general ill health, thirst, 'sighing' respiration, low temperature and blood pressure, rapid pulse, epigastric pain, smell of acetone: sugar and acetone in urine.

Hypoglycaemia ('insulin reaction', from excess of insulin) usually develops in minutes, with weakness, hunger, sweating, raised pulse: no sugar or acetone in urine.

Both hyperglycaemia and hypoglycaemia may lead to coma and death.

Treatment. Diet for all to regulate carbohydrate intake and reduce obesity. *Insulin for most:* soluble insulin (rapid action, given twice a day or mixed with long-acting preparation, e.g. protamine zinc insulin, P.Z.I.). Insulin zinc suspensions (semilente, lente, ultralente) may be mixed with each other but not with soluble insulin. Various other short and long-acting preparations. *Tablets*, e.g. tolbutamide or chlorpropamide, may control mild diabetics without insulin.

Hyperglycaemic coma or ketosis. Soluble insulin in large doses initially. Liberal intravenous saline. Electrolytes (especially potassium when recovering) according to deficiencies.

Hypoglycaemic coma. Glucose by mouth or intravenously. Sometimes adrenaline or glucagon. Adjust insulin dosage.

Care of feet to avoid septic ulcers and gangrene. Special treatment for other complications.

Special Tests. Test urine for sugar and acetone. Blood sugar estimation (fasting and at other times), for general control and in hyperglycaemia or hypoglycaemia. Glucose tolerance test. Serum electrolytes in hyperglycaemia.

Nursing Point. Detection of hypoglycaemia in patients in hospital relies on observant nurses: may occur at night.

Other points. Many elderly obese diabetics controlled by diet alone. Patient should be trained in measuring diet and giving insulin whilst in hospital. Patient lives many years with careful treatment. Infection may cause hyperglycaemic coma. Exercise may cause hypoglycaemia. Glycosuria may occur in other conditions besides diabetes, e.g. low renal glucose threshold, pregnancy. Steroid treatment or Cushing's syndrome may cause glycosuria and even diabetes. Diabetics undergoing surgery require close supervision: put on 4-hourly soluble insulin—dose determined by urine testing for sugar.

DIPHTHERIA

Condition. A specific infectious disease in which a membrane is present in the throat. Absorption of toxin causes symptoms in other organs.

Cause. Corynebacterium diphtheriae.

Occurrence. Usually children but adults may be attacked.

Incubation Period. Two to six days.

Symptoms and Signs. Malaise. Headache. Mild fever. Offensive breath. Sore throat, may be slight. Enlarged lymph nodes in neck. Adherent greyish-white membrane on throat. Laryngeal type: cough, hoarseness, stridor, cyanosis, recession of chest on respiration. Nasal type (mild): nasal discharge.

Complications. Myocarditis: fast or irregular pulse, pallor. Paralysis: palate, eyes, limbs, etc. Asphyxia in laryngeal type.

Treatment. Isolation. Antitoxin. Antibiotics. Antiseptic mouth-washes. Complete rest for several weeks. Laryngeal type—steam tent, tracheostomy if necessary.

May Resemble. Tonsillitis. Glandular Fever. Vincent's angina. Laryngitis. Foreign body in nose.

Special Tests. Throat swabs—will also detect healthy carriers. Schick test, shows those susceptible. E.C.G. if cardiac changes.

Nursing Points. Prevent all effort. Nurse flat, gradual pillows in convalescence. Glucose drinks. Disinfection of articles. Special measures in complications.

Other Points. Lasts six weeks, or longer if complications. Mortality low if treated early. 'Gravis' type causes more serious attack. Other sites may be affected: conjunctiva, wounds, vulva. May be carried in throat, nose or ear by convalescents or contacts. Negative swabs should be obtained before hospital discharge. Incidence very greatly reduced by immunization. Notifiable disease—notify Medical Officer of Health.

DISSEMINATED SCLEROSIS
(MULTIPLE SCLEROSIS)

Condition. A chronic relapsing disease in which demyelination occurs in scattered areas of the central nervous system.

Cause. Unknown.

Occurrence. Especially early adult life.

Symptoms and Signs. Early (tend to occur singly and briefly, but eventually accumulate and progress). Blurring of vision, diplopia, nystagmus. Weakness, stiffness or jerking of leg(s). Tremor on movement. Slurred speech. Pain, numbness, tingling. Bladder symptoms. *Later.* Spastic paralysis, ataxia, incontinence, emotional change. Bed sores, urinary infections, pneumonia.

Treatment. General hygiene. Reassurance and encouragement. Avoidance of fatigue. Physiotherapy, exercises. Orthopaedic appliances and operations. No specific treatment. Symptomatic treatment.

May Resemble. Other diseases of nervous system. Hysteria.

Special Test. Examination of cerebrospinal fluid.

Nursing Points. Keep patient active as long as possible. Special care in bed-ridden stage. Institutional care may be required.

Other Points. Course very variable. A very wide variety of neurological symptoms and signs may occur. A remission may last for years, or even occasionally be permanent, but average duration of life is about twenty years from onset.

DYSENTERY

Condition. Inflammation of the colon and rectum accompanied by diarrhoea.

Causes.

Bacillary—Shigella (Sonne, Shiga, Flexner).

Amoebic—Entamoeba histolytica.

Occurrence. Common abroad. Epidemics occur in this country, especially in institutions and camps.

Incubation Period. Bacillary 2 to 7 days. Amoebic may be months.

Symptoms and Signs. Griping pains. Diarrhoea, often with blood and mucus. Painful ineffectual defaecation ('tenesmus'). Fever. Abdominal tenderness. Loss of weight. Dehydration.

Complications. Amoebic: liver abscess and hepatitis.

Treatment. Bacillary—neomycin or sulphonamides, analgesics, correction of dehydration, antitoxin for Shiga group. Amoebic—emetine, bismuth iodide, chloroquine or metronidazole for hepatic complications.

May Resemble. Food poisoning. Appendicitis. Enteric fever. Cancer of colon or rectum.

Special Tests. Examination of fresh stools. Sigmoidoscopy (chronic cases).

Nursing Points. Warmth. Free fluids. Disposal of excreta.

Other Points. Varies greatly in severity. Bacillary type usually acute. Amoebic type may give chronic or intermittent symptoms. Carriers of both may have no symptoms. Prevention requires hygiene, detection of carriers, thorough cooking of food (and boiling of water, especially in tropics). Notifiable disease.

ECZEMA

Condition. A skin eruption, with erythema, vesicles and crusts.

Causes. Irritants (chemicals, discharges, light). Allergy (contact with or ingestion of substances, e.g. plants, drugs, clothing, cosmetics, detergents). Venous stasis and oedema (e.g. varicose veins—'varicose eczema'). Various general diseases; psychological factors.

Occurrence The commonest skin disease. Common at all ages from infancy upwards.

Distribution. Any part of skin: commonest on flexor aspects and face.

Course. Starts as erythema, then vesicles which 'weep' and may form crusts or scales. May last for months and liable to frequent recurrence. 'Varicose eczema' shows brownish areas liable to ulceration.

Treatment. Remove cause if known. Avoid scratching (gloves for child at night). Wet compresses and lotions if acute. Later, zinc or tar pastes, steroid preparations, etc. Sometimes antihistamines or sedatives. X-rays for some chronic types. Varicose eczema—elastic stocking or bandage, elevation of leg, surgical treatment of varicose veins.

Special Test. Patch tests for skin sensitivities.

Other Point. Basis may be an abnormal condition of the skin which may be hereditary (atopic eczema).

EMPHYSEMA

Condition. Progressive distension and destruction of lung alveoli.

Causes.
1. Pressure on lung alveoli by coughing and bronchospasm in chronic bronchitis and asthma (and destruction by infection and inflammation).
2. Compensatory dilatation in one part of lung due to collapse in another.
3. Degeneration in old age.

Occurrence. Middle and later life. Especially males.

Symptoms and Signs. Dyspnoea. Cyanosis. Barrel-shaped chest. Kyphosis. Poorly expanding hyper-resonant chest with poor breath sounds. Frequently signs of associated chronic bronchitis.

Complications. Chest infections. Heart failure. Pneumothorax.

Treatment. Limited activity. Warm climate if practicable. Treat any infection quickly. Correct malnutrition. Expectorants and bronchodilators. Oxygen if required. Breathing exercises (especially abdominal).

Special Tests. Chest X-ray. Sputum culture. Breathing tests. E.C.G.

Other Points. Slowly progressive, with decreasing exercise tolerance and eventually death from infection or heart failure. See also Chronic Bronchitis.

ENCEPHALITIS LETHARGICA
(EPIDEMIC ENCEPHALITIS)

Condition. An acute diffuse infection mainly of the lower brain.

Cause. Probably a virus.

Occurrence. Especially young adults. Often in epidemics (occurred between 1916 and 1926). Now rare but after-effects still seen.

Incubation Period. Seven to twenty-one days.

Symptoms and Signs. Acute stage. Headache. Inversion of sleep pattern; lethargy or confusion and restlessness. Blurred vision or diplopia and squint, ptosis. Sometimes fever, delirium, convulsions. *Later.* Parkinsonism. Nervousness, depression, etc. (sometimes severe mental changes and anti-social behaviour, especially in children). Involuntary movements. Disturbances of sleep and vision may persist. Oculogyric crises—see under Parkinsonism.

Course. May be fatal, recover at any stage, arrest with residual symptoms, or be slowly progressive. Now usually mild disease, but in earlier epidemics 20 to 40 per cent died.

Treatment. General measures. Sedatives. Disinfect discharges and excretions.

May Resemble. Poliomyelitis. Meningitis. Botulism. Other causes of coma and Parkinsonism.

Special Test. Lumbar puncture to exclude meningitis, etc.

Other Points. Notifiable disease. Called 'sleepy sickness'; but distinguish from 'sleeping sickness'—trypanosomiasis. Other forms of encephalitis occur occasionally in measles, mumps, smallpox and other virus diseases.

ENDOCARDITIS (SUB-ACUTE BACTERIAL)

Condition. Infection of the endocardium over an abnormal heart valve by 'non-pathogenic' bacteria (i.e. bacteria which would cause no harm to normal valves). 'Vegetations' form on valves.

Cause. Bacteraemia: especially release into blood of Streptococcus viridans from teeth, by dental extractions or filling, or chewing. Sometimes organisms from other septic foci.

Occurrence. Especially young adults.

Symptoms and Signs. Persistent fever. Sweating. Malaise or fatigue. Sometimes joint pains. New heart murmurs. Anaemia. Splenomegaly. Emboli (from vegetations breaking off valves): skin—splinter haemorrhages under nails, tender nodules on hands and feet, petechiae; spleen—pain in left side; kidney—haematuria; brain—signs of cerebrovascular accident. Later, finger clubbing, cachexia, 'café-au-lait' complexion.

Complication. The valves are further damaged; may produce heart failure.

Treatment. Bed rest. Penicillin (or appropriate antibiotic)—large doses for several weeks.

May Resemble. Other causes of persistent fever and malaise. Miliary tuberculosis. Typhoid. Embolism resembles other disease of organs involved.

Special Tests. Blood cultures. E.S.R. Blood count. Microscopy of urine for red cells.

Nursing Point. Long hospital stay produces boredom and depression, especially since patient feels fairly fit after starting treatment.

Other Points. Avoid by penicillin cover of oral surgery in patients with known heart valve disease. A common cause of 'P.U.O.' (pyrexia of unknown origin). Previous heart disease may be unknown. Most recover with antibiotics, but residual damage common. Other forms of endocarditis: 1. Acute—

invasion of normal valves by virulent bacteria (but rare since antibiotics introduced). 2. Rheumatic—see under Rheumatic Fever.

ENURESIS (NOCTURNAL)

Condition. Bedwetting.

Causes. Usually emotional insecurity. Fear of punishment. Perhaps mental deficiency. Sometimes disease of urinary tract or spinal cord, diabetes mellitus or diabetes insipidus.

Occurrence. Young children, especially boys. May persist to puberty.

Symptoms and Signs. Wetting the bed at night. May be frequency in daytime.

Treatment. If cause is emotional, encouragement of warmer relationship between parents and child; psychotherapy if necessary. Restrict evening fluids. Empty bladder at bedtime and perhaps during night. Encourage when dry and do not blame when wet. Controlled micturition and bladder exercises by day, to train bladder. Belladonna. Electrical warning arrangements. Tricyclic antidepressants.

EPILEPSY

Condition. Periodic transitory disorder of cerebral function with changes of consciousness.

Causes. Idiopathic ('constitutional')—usually starts in childhood and may be hereditary. Infantile convulsions. Congenital brain disease. Head injury. Meningitis. Tumour. Arterial degeneration. Stokes-Adams attacks. Metabolic disturbance (e.g. uraemia, hypoglycaemia). Anoxia (e.g. respiratory failure). Poisons. Neurosyphilis.

Special Test. Electro-encephalogram (E.E.G.)

Other Points. Most cases controlled satisfactorily by drugs. Severe cases require institutional treatment. Attacks may occur during sleep. Find suitable employment. Forbid car driving. Protect open fires. Pregnancy may worsen attacks.

GRAND MAL or MAJOR EPILEPSY

Symptoms and Signs. May have preliminary 'aura' (noises or other sensations). Then unconsciousness: *tonic stage*, general rigidity, may be cyanosis, lasts a few seconds; *clonic stage*, twitching followed by convulsive movements, biting of tongue, micturition, frothing at mouth; *coma*, body flaccid; often passes into sleep or drowsiness. Following a fit may be 'automatism' (actions performed without later remembrance), or 'status epilepticus' (continued recurrence of fits without recovery of consciousness, serious). Automatism may be pleaded as a defence in some criminal cases.

Complications. Injuries during fit. Mental deterioration.

Treatment. Regular life. Avoid alcohol, excessive fluid intake and violent exercise. Phenobarbitone. Phenytoin. Primidone. Treat cause. Status epilepticus: diazepam, paraldehyde or barbiturates intramuscularly or intravenously.

Nursing Points. During attack remove false teeth, place gag between teeth. Keep tongue forward. Loosen clothing. Turn on side if vomiting.

JACKSONIAN EPILEPSY

Cause. Usually organic brain disease, e.g. tumours, injuries.

Symptoms and Signs. Localized movement starting in part of a limb, often without loss of consciousness. May remain localized or may spread slowly to surrounding parts of body. May progress to grand mal.

Treatment. As in grand mal.

PETIT MAL or MINOR EPILEPSY

Cause. Always idiopathic ('constitutional').

Symptoms and Signs. Short loss of consciousness without convulsion. Often staring expression. Action being performed suddenly interrupted and then continued after attack. May be followed by 'automatism'. Frequent such attacks—'pyknolepsy'.

Treatment. Ethosuximide. Troxidone.

Other Point. Usually in children.

TEMPORAL LOBE or PSYCHOMOTOR EPILEPSY

Symptoms and Signs. Hallucinations or vivid emotions or memories, with automatic unconscious actions—smacking lips, undressing, etc. Occasionally ends in grand mal convulsions.

Treatment. Phenytoin. Primidone. Surgical removal of lesion in temporal lobe occasionally possible. (With other forms of epilepsy due to lesions elsewhere, surgery would usually cause too much damage to be practicable.)

ERYSIPELAS

Condition. An acute infection of the skin.

Cause. Haemolytic streptococcus.

Occurrence. Any age. Commoner in latter half of life and in ill health.

Incubation period. 1 to 7 days.

Symptoms and Signs. Headache. Malaise. Fever. Vomiting. Rash on first day, spreading area of erythema with raised edges, hot and tender. Spreads fast for a few days. Vesicles and bullae appear later. Abrasion or wound, where organism entered, may be present. Face commonest site.

Complications. Delirium. Septicamia. Cellulitis and abscess formation. Meningitis (if scalp affected). Nephritis. Bronchopneumonia.

Treatment. Penicillin. Sedatives.

May Resemble. Cellulitis.

Nursing Points. Local applications to area. Covering not always necessary. Bathing of eyes if face affected. Watch for delirium.

Other Points. Usually recovers rapidly if treated early. Notifiable disease.

ERYTHEMA NODOSUM

Condition. Reddish swellings usually on the front of the legs.

Causes. May be associated with drugs (especially sulphonamides) or infectious or other diseases, e.g. tuberculosis, sarcoidosis, rheumatic fever, streptococcal infections, ulcerative colitis, some venereal diseases.

Occurrence. Chiefly in young adult females.

Symptoms and Signs. Oval or round, dark red, tender swellings, about 1 cm in diameter. Sometimes fever, malaise, joint pain. Also features of causative disease.

Treatment. Bed rest if severe. Soothing applications to areas. Treat underlying disease.

Special Tests. Chest X-ray. E.S.R. Throat swab. Mantoux and Kweim tests.

Prognosis. Disappears over a matter of weeks.

FOOD POISONING

Condition. An acute disease with gastro-intestinal symptoms due to infected, contaminated or poisonous food.

Causes. Food usually contaminated during distribution or preparation. Inadequate cooking or refrigeration. Occasionally poisonous fungi (toadstools) or chemicals.

Symptoms and Signs. Usually arise within 24 hours. Malaise. Headache. Abdominal pain and diarrhoea. Vomiting.

Treatment. Warmth. Fluids freely—intravenously if necessary. Kaolin. Perhaps antibiotics. Perhaps stomach wash-out.

May Resemble. Appendicitis. Dysentery. Typhoid.

Special Tests. Examination of stools, vomit and food concerned if available. Blood agglutination reactions.

Other Points. Several people often affected at same time. May be a carrier infecting food. Chiefly arises from meat. May be produced by live organisms (especially Salmonellae) entering gut, or by toxin produced by bacteria in food before eating (especially Staphylococci; this type is therefore not prevented by subsequent cooking and not treatable by antibiotics). Mortality low except in massive infection. Notifiable disease.

OTHER TYPES OF FOOD POISONING

Allergy. Certain individuals are unduly sensitive to certain foods, and may develop gastro-enteritis and urticaria after eating eggs, shellfish, etc.

Botulism. Due to eating food infected with B. botulinus (may occur with canned foods, pastes, pasties, sausages). Causes nausea, headache, dizziness, ocular paralyses (double vision, etc.), difficulty in swallowing, respiratory troubles. Mortality often high. Very rare.

Note. Some other diseases may be spread by food, e.g. dysentery, typhoid, cholera, tuberculosis.

GASTRITIS (ACUTE)

Condition. Acute inflammation of the stomach.

Causes. Irritating food or drink. Poisons. Infections.

Symptoms and Signs. Anorexia. Nausea. Vomiting. Abdominal pain. Weakness. Thirst.

Treatment. Warmth. Perhaps stomach washout. Warm fluids. Milk diet. Antidote, if poison. Treat diarrhoea if present.

Other Points. May occur with ulcer, enteritis, diarrhoea. May occur at onset of an infectious disease, especially influenza Aspirin is a common cause of massive blood loss.

GASTRITIS (CHRONIC)

Condition. Chronic inflammation of the stomach with mucosal atrophy.

Cause. Indefinite.

Symptoms and Signs. Symptoms either absent, or like those of peptic ulcer.

Complications. Gastric bleeding. Pernicious anaemia and gastric carcinoma are associated with gastric atrophy, possibly caused by it.

Treatment. Regular life. Suitable diet (exclude rich foods). Attention to teeth. Perhaps stop smoking and alcohol. Perhaps ulcer therapy. Treat anaemia and carcinoma.

May Resemble. Peptic ulcer. Carcinoma of stomach.

Special Tests. Histamine test (acid low or absent). Barium meal. Gastroscopy.

Other Points. 'Nervous dyspepsia' is a form of indigestion associated with disordered function of a nervous type. See also Irritable Colon, Anorexia Nervosa.

GASTRO-ENTERITIS (INFANTILE)

Condition. An acute infection causing diarrhoea and vomiting.

Causes. Usually infection conveyed through milk, especially E. coli. Flies and lack of hygiene.

Occurrence. Especially in children under two years and in bottle-fed infants. Overcrowding. Poverty. Malnutrition. Commonest in late summer months ('summer diarrhoea'). Much less common since improvements in hygiene and milk preparation.

Symptoms and Signs. Listless. Diarrhoea. Foul, frequent, greenish stools. Vomiting. Dehydration. Acidosis. Usually fever and shock.

Treatment. Intravenous fluids controlled by serum electrolyte estimations. Starve at first, then gradual return to full diet. Neomycin and other antibiotics.

Special Tests. Microscopy and culture of faeces.

Nursing Points. Isolation. Fresh air. Pasteurization of milk. Boiling of water. Scrupulous cleanliness and avoidance of transfer of infection. Keep mouth clean. Disinfection of infected linen.

Other Points. Mortality low if the infant previously healthy, but high when other disease present, or in the neglected child. Attend to elimination of and protection from flies. Highly infectious: may become epidemic in nurseries.

GOITRE

Condition. Enlargement of thyroid gland.
Causes.

1. Thyrotoxicosis.
2. Simple (colloid or endemic) goitre: iodine deficiency.

3. Hashimoto's or other forms of thyroiditis.
4. Thyroid adenoma or carcinoma.

Occurrence. Simple goitre occurs especially in districts with little iodine in water (e.g. Derbyshire).

Symptoms and Signs. Swelling in neck. All types occasionally produce pressure symptoms (especially if large retrosternal extension): venous congestion, dysphagia, dyspnoea. *Special features:* of 1—see Thyrotoxicosis; of 2—occasionally Myxoedema; of 3—often Myxoedema; of 4—carcinoma often produces hoarseness (due to invasion of recurrent laryngeal nerve) and metastases to lymph nodes or elsewhere.

Treatment. For 1, see under Thyrotoxicosis. For 2, potassium iodide, thyroxine, partial thyroidectomy. For 3, thyroxine. For 4, removal or radiotherapy.

Special Tests. X-ray thoracic inlet. Radioactive iodine uptake of gland, plasma protein-bound iodine. Tests of pituitary control. Occasionally, biopsy.

Prognosis. Thyroid carcinoma may be rapidly fatal. Other types can usually be well controlled.

GONORRHOEA

Condition. An acute venereal infection of the urinary and genital tracts.

Cause. Gonococcus.

Occurrence. Chiefly young adults.

Mode of Infection. Genital contact with infected person. Infection of newborn's eyes from mother, or vulvo-vaginitis in infants.

Incubation period. About 3 to 10 days.

Symptoms. Male: acute purulent discharge from urethra.

Female: over 50 per cent have no symptoms. May have vaginal discharge. Both may have dysuria and frequency.

Complications. Male: epididymitis, prostatitis, later urethral stricture, occasional sterility. Distant lesions (arthritis) very rare. Female: Bartholin's abscess, salpingitis, peritonitis, sterility.

Treatment. Penicillin or other antibiotics in appropriate doses. Special treatment of complications.

Special Tests. Male: microscopy and culture of urethral or rectal discharge (in passive homosexuals). Female: microscopy and culture of cervical, urethral and rectal specimens. Complement fixation test (G.C.F.T.) not used as inaccurate.

Other Points. Can be completely cured if treated early and thoroughly. Gonococci difficult to find in discharge if patient has already received drug therapy; fluorescent slides may help. Also there may be coexistent syphilis and/or trichomoniasis. Number of cases of venereal disease has increased in last few years. Reiter's syndrome consists of urethritis, arthritis, conjunctivitis, not caused by gonococcus, and not always related to sexual intercourse. Ophthalmia neonatorum is a notifiable disease.

GOUT

Condition. A type of recurrent acute arthritis.

Cause. Inborn error of metabolism. Urate crystals deposited in region of joints. In susceptible people, attack may be precipitated by alcohol, certain foods, injury, surgery, infections, diuretic drugs. Occurs also in treatment of acute luekaemia, due to increased cell turnover.

Occurrence. Middle-aged men (very rare in women). Often hereditary.

Symptoms and Signs. Malaise. Sudden attack of intense pain in joint, often at night. Joint swollen and tender with red shiny appearance. Joints chiefly affected: big toes (commonest), ankles, knees, fingers. Often fever. After some years, tophi (chalky deposits of urates) in ears, knuckles, etc.

Complications. Osteoarthritis. Chronic renal failure. Renal stones. Hypertension.

Treatment. Acute attack—high fluid intake, analgesics, colchicine, phenylbutazone, A.C.T.H. *Chronic gout*—exclude factors precipitating attacks, high fluid intake, allopurinol (reduces formation of uric acid) for life, and physiotherapy. Treat complications.

May Resemble. Other types of arthritis.

Special Tests. Blood uric acid (raised). X-ray joints.

Nursing Points. Remember joints are acutely painful. Wrap in wool. Hot applications. Cradle over joints.

Other Points. Attacks occur with increasing frequency, and persistent pain may develop with stiff, deformed joints. Prognosis for life is usually good, unless hypertension and arterial degeneration occur.

HAEMOLYTIC DISEASE OF NEWBORN
(ICTERUS GRAVIS NEONATORUM; ERYTHROBLASTOSIS FOETALIS)

Condition. Haemolytic anaemia, often severe with jaundice, due to destruction of infant's red cells by antibodies from mother.

Cause. Usually presence of Rhesus factor in infant's red cells and absence in mother's.

Occurrence. Signs appear a few hours or days after birth.

Symptoms and Signs. Jaundice. Severe anaemia. Enlargement of liver and spleen. Occasionally haemorrhage.

Complications. Kernicterus—brain damage causing lethargy and spasms of rigidity and other disorders—dangerous. Intrauterine death.

Special Tests. Blood film and count. Direct Coombs' test positive. Serum bilirubin raised. Maternal blood for antibodies (rising level during pregnancy indicates necessity for hospital confinement).

Treatment. Exchange transfusion of blood of suitable type.

Other Points. Rarely in ABO incompatibility. Not in first pregnancy, unless mother has been transfused with Rhesus positive blood. Likelihood and severity increase with further pregnancies, eventually producing foetal death. Prognosis varies, but most make complete recovery with treatment. Kernicterus may leave permanent brain damage. Totally preventable by using Anti-D globulin in susceptible mothers.

HAEMORRHAGIC DISEASE OF NEWBORN

Condition. Abnormal bleeding in newborn.

Causes. Low blood level of prothrombin (and other factors): prothrombin synthesis not yet fully established in neonatal liver. Various other bleeding diseases are an occasional cause.

Occurrence. Between 2nd and 5th days of life. Especially if premature.

Symptoms and Signs. Bleeding from gastro-intestinal tract (melaena or haematemesis), nose, umbilical cord stump, renal tract (haematuria), vagina, brain (irritability, convulsions or coma), or lungs (rapid suffocation). Pallor, tachycardia and shock if severe.

Treatment. Vitamin K_1 (may be given prophylactically in prematurity: also after abnormal deliveries, because of likelihood of trauma). Blood transfusion if severe.

Special Tests. Haemoglobin. Bleeding, clotting and prothrombin times. Distinguish mother's from infant's haemoglobin (see *Other Points*).

Other Points. Majority recover and have no further bleeding tendencies. Bleeding into lungs or brain sometimes fatal. Normal infant's stools or vomit may contain blood swallowed during delivery, but not beyond 24 hours after birth.

HEART BLOCK

Condition. Interference with conduction between atria and ventricles (in Bundle of His). If '2nd degree' (partial), ventricles contract with every 2nd (or 3rd or 4th) atrial contraction. If '3rd degree' (complete), ventricles contract independently of atria (and slower).

Causes. Ischaemia. Active rheumatic fever or diphtheria. Drug excess—digitalis, quinidine. Occasionally congenital or syphilitic.

Occurrence. Commoner in males.

Symptoms and Signs. Arterial pulse (30-50): slower than venous. Venous 'cannon waves' in neck in complete type. Symptoms of causative disease.

Complications. 'Stokes-Adams' attacks: episodes of unconsciousness (perhaps with convulsions) resulting from stopping or extreme slowness of heart beat.

Treatment. Avoid excessive exertion. Treat cause. If liable to 'Stokes-Adams' attacks: isoprenaline, ephedrine, perhaps steroids in acute cases: surgically implanted electrical pacemakers: in a severe attack, external cardiac massage and D.C. shock.

Special Tests. E.C.G. Chest X-ray.

Other Points. Congenital type may be benign, but in other types death usually occurs within a few years, especially if 'Stokes-Adams' attacks occur.

HEART FAILURE

Condition. Heart is unable to maintain an adequate circulation of blood. May be acute or chronic, or left or right side of heart (usually both).

Causes. Left-sided: ischaemic heart disease; hypertension; rheumatic heart disease; other valvular disease (congenital, syphilitic, etc.); congenital heart disease; thyrotoxicosis; myxoedema; anaemia; myocardial degeneration; terminal stage of many illnesses. *Right-sided:* failure is usually secondary to left-sided, but may be due to chest diseases (then called 'cor pulmonale'), especially emphysema, pulmonary embolism.

Symptoms and Signs. Fatigue. Increased heart size, sometimes abnormal heart sounds. Sometimes pleural effusion. *Left-sided:* dyspnoea—at first on exercise: then on lying down ('orthopnoea') or in middle of night ('paroxysmal nocturnal dyspnoea'): later, present all the time. Cough—pink, frothy sputum or haemoptysis. Cold, cyanosed extremities. Cerebral anoxia (confusion, Cheyne-Stokes respiration). Pulsus alternans. On auscultation, crepitations in lungs. *Right-sided:* Oedema. Distended neck veins. Enlarged liver (sometimes cirrhosis later). Ascites. Diminished urine. Anorexia.

Treatment. Rest. Prop up. Digitalis. Diuretics. Restrict salt intake. Treat cause if possible. Removal of pleural or ascitic fluids (and occasionally of subcutaneous fluid by Southey's tubes). In acute left-sided failure (e.g. 'paroxysmal nocturnal dyspnoea')—morphia, oxygen, aminophylline: occasionally venous cuffs on thighs, venesection.

Special Tests. E.C.G. X-ray chest. Measure fluid intake and output. Blood count, blood urea and electrolytes.

Nursing Points. Nurse upright in bed with bed-table for support. Anticipate every effort. Encourage leg movements and avoid pillow behind knees, to prevent leg-vein thrombosis. Care of skin. Accurate fluid chart. Watch for toxic effects of digitalis—slow pulse, coupled beats, nausea, vomiting. Watch for night restlessness. Tight binder after tapping ascites.

HERPES ZOSTER
(SHINGLES)

Condition. A vesicular eruption in the area of distribution of a sensory nerve.

Cause. Virus affecting the posterior root ganglion of the spinal cord. The same virus causes chicken-pox.

Symptoms and Signs. May be pyrexia and malaise. Pain in the affected area followed by an eruption of papules which later became vesicular. Common areas: trunk, face. Usually unilateral.

Treatment. Analgesics. Antiseptic dusting powders or lotions. Antibiotics if secondarily infected. Steroids in the elderly.

Other Points. Occasionally followed by persistent post-herpetic pain (especially in elderly). Herpes-like rash occurring on lips in other infections, e.g. pneumonia, is a different type—'herpes simplex'.

HODGKIN'S DISEASE
(LYMPHADENOMA)

Condition. Malignant tumour of lymphoid tissue.

Cause. Not known.

Occurrence. Usually young adults. Commoner in males.

Symptoms and signs. Insidious progressive enlargement of cervical, axillary, inguinal, mediastinal and mesenteric lymph nodes—often starting in cervical. Nodes are painless and rubbery. Enlarged spleen and liver. Fatigue, malaise, sweats. Pressure signs in mediastinum (see under Mediastinal Obstruction), bones, spinal cord, abdomen, etc. Fever may be low-grade, irregular or 'Pel-Ebstein' type—raised temperature for some days, alternating with normal temperature for some days. Anaemia. Alcoholic drinks may cause pain in involved nodes.

Treatment. Radiotherapy. Combination cytotoxic chemotherapy in special centre. Steroids. Treatment of symptoms.

May Resemble. Other causes of enlarged lymph nodes—malignant growths, leukaemia, chronic infection, tuberculosis, sarcoidosis, infectious mononucleosis.

Special Tests Biopsy of node. Blood count (variable—anaemia, eosinophils increased, etc.). E.S.R. Bone marrow examination.

Other Points. Fatal disease: may last a few months or many years, but prognosis is greatly improved—average 2 or 3 years. Hodgkin's is the commonest of the reticuloses or malignant lymphomas: others are follicular lymphoma (or lymphoid follicular reticulosis) which is less rapidly fatal, and lymphosarcoma and reticulum cell sarcoma, which are more rapidly fatal.

HYPERTENSION

Condition. High blood pressure.

Causes. In most cases, of unknown cause with hereditary factor ('essential hypertension')—obesity and mental stress are possible factors. Sometimes due to renal or arterial disease, toxaemia of pregnancy, or endocrine disorders (e.g. Cushing's syndrome or steroid treatment).

Symptoms and Signs. Usually none at first, except high blood pressure: often found on routine medical examination. Later, the features of the complications.

Complications. Enlarged heart. Heart failure. Arterial Degeneration and its complications (especially cerebral haemorrhage and ischaemic heart disease). Retinopathy: haemorrhages, etc., in optic fundus may impair sight; papilloedema in 'malignant hypertension'. Chronic renal disease with albuminuria. Occasionally 'hypertensive encephalopathy' (convulsions or other cerebral disorders): especially with rapid rise of pressure, e.g. in acute nephritis or eclampsia.

Treatment. Avoid obesity and strenuous exertion. Reassurance and sometimes sedatives. Find suitable job. Hypotensive drugs which prevent vasoconstriction, by acting on the brain, sympathetic nerves or arteries (e.g. reserpine, methyl dopa, guanethidine, bethanidine, guanoxan). Thiazide diuretics.

Complications of Treatment. Hypotensive drugs may produce dizziness or fainting on standing up (since many act mainly when standing), dry mouth, blocked nose, constipation or diarrhoea, impotence, urinary retention, paralysis of lens accommodation, fluid retention, depression, drowsiness or tremor. Excessive reduction of blood pressure may produce cerebral or coronary thrombosis or renal failure.

Special Tests. E.C.G. Blood urea. Urine culture and examination. X-ray chest. Intravenous pyelogram (I.V.P.) (or isotope renogram or occasionally renal arteriogram).

Nursing Point. Take blood pressure regularly, lying and standing.

Other Points. Occasional high reading may occur in normal people, especially in excitement or exercise. Raised diastolic pressure often more important than raised systolic pressure. Life expectancy is reduced, especially in young men with high diastolic pressures.

HYSTERIA

Condition. Symptoms and signs often imitating organic disease, but of psychological origin (arising subconsciously—in contrast to malingering).

Occurrence. Commoner in females, especially adolescents and young adults. Usually in hysterical type of personality.

Symptoms and Signs. May be any clinical picture.

Motor Signs. Paralysis. Loss of voice. Spasmodic movements. Fits (occur in presence of others: no injuries or micturition). Hyperventilation, leading to tetany and tingling.

Sensory. Areas of pain or anaesthesia. Palate may be anaesthetic (no gag reflex) in hysteria in contrast to malingering. Partial loss of vision.

Psychological. Amnesia. Stupor.

Treatment. Psychiatric investigation and treatment: sudden cure may result. Change of environment, remove patient from too sympathetic relatives or friends. Suitable work. When acute symptoms disappear treat underlying personality or situation.

May Resemble. Organic diseases.

Special Tests. Those of the organic disease simulated.

Nursing Points. Do not blame patient. Understanding attitude without pampering.

Other Points. Large variety of symptoms may occur. Absence of certain symptoms and signs which would be present in organic disease, e.g. area of anaesthesia may not correspond with anatomical nerve distribution. May come on after an emotional upset. Hysterical symptoms may arise in addition to an organic disease being present. Hysteria is one type of neurotic manifestation: see under Neurosis.

IMPETIGO CONTAGIOSA

Condition. A pustular infection of the skin. Contagious.
Causes. Staphylococci (occasionally streptococci).
Occurrence. Very common especially in poor children.
Distribution. Chiefly affects face and scalp. Bullous vesicles become pustular with crusts. Spreads rapidly by scratching.
Treatment. Remove crusts gently with warm water. Antibiotic ointments (especially neomycin or Fucidin).
Nursing Points. Prevent scratching. Shave scalp. Individual utensils. Disinfection of clothing and bedding.
Other Points. Often associated with scabies or with discharge from nose or ear. 'Sycosis barbae' is a type of impetigo in men affecting the beard and moustache area.

INDUSTRIAL AND OCCUPATIONAL DISEASES

ACCIDENTS

These are the commonest cause of loss of working days. They can be reduced by protection of workers by special clothing, masks, guards on dangerous machines, and by adaptation of working conditions to eliminate fumes and dusts. Factories are required by law to conform to minimum standards of safety, and are inspected regularly. Workers should be instructed in the safe use of their equipment, as one of the commonest causes of accidents is failure to use the safeguards supplied.

CARCINOMA OF THE BLADDER

Cause. Exposure to aniline dyes, as in the rubber industry.

Symptoms and Signs. Haematuria or unexplained urinary tract infection in a patient who was exposed to the dyes often many years before the onset of symptoms.

Treatment. Diathermy under cystoscopic control, sometimes cystectomy or radiotherapy.

Other points. Persons known to have been exposed to the dyes in the past or at present should be examined routinely for haematuria.

FARMER'S LUNG

Condition. An allergic condition of the lung due to inhalation of spores in mouldy hay.

Cause. A fungus.

Symptoms and Signs. Fever, shortness of breath and bloodstained sputum, occurring in attacks, leading to progressive respiratory and cardiac failure.

Treatment. Steroids in the acute attack. Careful farming. Often change of occupation.

LEAD POISONING (ACUTE OR CHRONIC)

Causes. Usually due to chronic ingestion of lead from air, food or water.

Symptoms and Signs. Usually present with neurological damage: wrist drop or psychiatric changes in adults. Children may present with skin rashes, anaemia or failure to thrive.

Special tests. Blood film. Urinary lead excretion.

Treatment. Chelating blood (EDTA). Removal of cause of poisoning.

Other Points. Children may eat lead-containing paint in old houses, and this is particularly common in immigrant children. Lead-based paints should never be used. May occur in lead smelters, painters, pottery glazers and the motor industry.

PNEUMOCONIOSIS

Condition. Chronic inflammation and fibrosis of the lungs following inhalation of various dusts.

Causes. Long exposure to dusts of various types—coal, silica, stone, asbestos, etc.

Occurrence. Males working in special industries.

Symptoms and Signs. No symptoms at first. Increasing dyspnoea. Later, cough. Chronic bronchitis often associated.

Complications. Pulmonary tuberculosis very common. Emphysema. Cor pulmonale (right-sided heart failure). Bronchial carcinoma and finger clubbing, especially in asbestosis.

Treatment. Change of employment. Treat complications.

Special Tests. X-ray: fine, later coarse, shadows in lungs. Examine sputum.

Other Points. Gradual deterioration over 10 to 20 years (longer with coal miners), to death from complications. Special factory regulations have reduced the number of cases: dust extractors, wet methods, respirators, washing of hands, etc. Special names are given to the various types, e.g. silicosis (silica), anthracosis (coal). Some other dusts, e.g. iron, produce X-ray shadows but no symptoms or lung damage. These industrial diseases qualify for compensation.

INFECTIOUS MONONUCLEOSIS
(GLANDULAR FEVER)

Condition. An infectious disease characterized by general malaise and swelling of lymph nodes.

Cause. Probably due to a virus.

Occurrence. Chiefly children and young adults.

Incubation Period. About 4 to 10 days.

Symptoms and Signs. Malaise. Fever. Sore throat. A few days later—enlarged lymph nodes. Enlargement of spleen. Sometimes a rash. May be jaundice.

Complications. Mild hepatitis common, occasionally with jaundice. Many other rare complications including rupture of spleen.

Treatment. Treatment of symptoms. Generous convalescence.

May Resemble. Other causes of enlarged lymph nodes or sore throat—tonsillitis, diphtheria, Hodgkin's disease, etc. Infectious hepatitis.

Special Tests. Blood count (monocytic cells increased, atypical lymphocytes present). Paul-Bunnell blood test. Liver function tests.

Other Points. Acute disease lasts about two weeks, but fatigue, depression and other symptoms may persist for months. Eventually, recovery is nearly always complete.

INFLUENZA

Condition. Highly infectious disease with pyrexia and symptoms chiefly of the respiratory or gastro-intestinal tracts.

Cause. Virus—influenza A or B.

Occurrence. Frequent epidemics, occasionally affecting large numbers with a considerable number of deaths. Commoner in winter.

Incubation Period. A few days.

Symptoms and Signs. Headache. Fever. Shivering. Sweating. Coryza. Cough. Anorexia. Muscular aching. Sometimes sore throat or vomiting.

Complications. Secondary infection. Broncho-pneumonia. Sinusitis. Depression.

Treatment. Aspirin. Symptomatic (bed rest, hot drinks). Special treatment of complications.

Other Points. Leads to short-lived specific immunity. Vaccine therapy in epidemics of some use. Many other presumably viral infections are often incorrectly called influenza.

IRRITABLE COLON

VARIETIES

Spastic Colon, Mucous Colitis, Nervous Diarrhoea, etc.

Condition. Group of disorders of colonic function, without organic disease or inflammation.

Causes. Obscure. Psychological factors, previous infections and dietary sensitivities contribute.

Symptoms and Signs. Any combination of diarrhoea, constipation, or abdominal pain, often intermittent. May pass mucus.

Treatment. Reassurance. Phenobarbitone, propantheline ('Pro-Banthine') and hydrophilic preparations (e.g. 'Normacol', 'Isogel', 'Celevac'). Codeine for diarrhoea.

May Resemble. Many other causes of recurrent abdominal symptoms, e.g. peptic ulcer, cholecystitis, appendicitis, ulcerative colitis, or carcinoma of stomach, pancreas, colon or of rectum.

ISCHAEMIC HEART DISEASE

Condition. Inadequate blood supply to heart muscle.

Causes. Coronary artery disease—see Arterial Degeneration; also occasionally anaemia, aortic aneurysm, syphilis.

Occurrence. Especially males beyond middle age. Common in professional classes.

Symptoms and Signs. Sudden tight pain in chest, often radiating to left arm, neck or epigastrium. Anxiety. Sometimes dyspnoea. Sometimes shock (hypotension, pallor, sweating). In myocardial infarction, also fever and sometimes heart failure.

Types—1. 'Angina pectoris': caused by exercise (or meal or emotion—increasing heart's work), relieved by rest.
2. 'Myocardial infarction' (='cardiac infarction' = 'coronary thrombosis'): not relieved by rest.

Treatment. Avoid excessive exertion. General treatment as for Arterial Degeneration.

Special Treatment.

1. Angina—treat attacks with rest, trinitrin (dissolve under tongue), occasionally morphia.
2. Myocardial infarction—lay flat. Morphia, oxygen. Lignocaine, sometimes atropine for arrhythmias. Digitalis if heart failure. Cardiac massage if cardiac arrest. Bed rest. Perhaps anticoagulants—heparin or phenindione ('Dindevan'), dosage of latter controlled by estimating prothrombin time.

May Resemble. Pulmonary embolism. Dissecting aneurysm. Acute abdominal condition (see under Cholecystitis).

Special Tests. E.C.G. Serum enzymes raised (e.g. S.G.O.T.). X-ray of heart.

Other Points. Myocardial infarction often fatal. If not, sometimes followed by angina pectoris, atrial fibrillation, heart failure or second infarction; but recovery to reduced or fairly normal activity often occurs.

JAUNDICE

Condition. Yellow pigmentation of skin and conjunctiva, due to raised serum bilirubin level.

Causes. Haemolytic. Hepatocellular. Obstructive.

Symptoms and Signs. Pruritus (itching) common with deep jaundice from any cause. Bleeding tendency (bruises, petechiae, prolonged bleeding after surgery), common with hepatocellular or obstructive: prothrombin time prolonged (i.e. reduced if reported as percentage).

Special Tests. Urine—bilirubin present in obstructive, urobilinogen increased in haemolytic, variable in hepatocellular. Serum bilirubin. Blood count to exclude haemolysis. Prothrombin time. Liver function tests: alkaline phosphatase (slightly raised in hepatocellular, greatly in obstructive); plasma proteins and serum electrophoresis (various abnormalities); serum transaminases especially S.G.P.T. (raised in liver damage). Plain X-ray for gall-stones. Liver biopsy occasionally.

JAUNDICE—HAEMOLYTIC
(ACHOLURIC)

Condition. Jaundice and anaemia and usually enlargement of spleen.

Cause. Haemolytic anaemia causing excessive destruction of red cells with increased bilirubin production.

Occurrence. See section on Haemolytic Anaemia.

Symptoms and Signs. Jaundice usually mild. Anaemia. Enlarged spleen common. No pain or pruritus. Pigment gallstones may be present. Crisis may occur—see under Haemolytic Anaemia.

Treatment. That of haemolytic anaemia.

Special Tests. Those of haemolytic anaemia. Liver function tests normal.

Other Points. Jaundice may be absent in haemolytic anaemia.

JAUNDICE—HEPATOCELLULAR

Condition. Liver cell damage due to infection or poisons.

Causes. Viruses of infective hepatitis and homologous serum jaundice. Weil's disease. Yellow Fever. Septicaemia. Poisons, e.g. carbon tetrachloride, chloroform, phosphorus. Acute yellow atrophy of liver. Cirrhosis.

Symptoms and Signs. Vary with cause. General symptoms often appear 1 to 4 days before jaundice. Features of renal, neurological or cardiac disease also present with Weil's disease and some poisons.

INFECTIVE HEPATITIS

Incubation Period. About 2 to 8 weeks.

Symptoms and Signs. Extreme anorexia. Often vomiting, headache and fever. Tender, enlarged liver and sometimes spleen. Jaundice after 3 or 4 days. Fever and pulse fall (often bradycardia). Pale stools, dark urine.

Treatment. No specific therapy. Bed rest. Diet: low fat often preferred; high calorie as soon as tolerated; no protein in severe case.

Special Tests. Liver function tests—abnormal, see above. Urine: bilirubin present throughout disease; urobilinogen present early and when recovery begins—absent in interval because intra-hepatic obstruction occurs.

Other Points. Epidemics occur. Most infectious before

jaundice appears. Isolation unnecessary but prevent spread. Great majority recover in 2 to 6 weeks: a few die in acute phase. Cirrhosis a rare complication. *Homologous serum jaundice* is similar disease with incubation period of about 8 to 26 weeks: virus transmitted through imperfectly sterilized needles or syringes, or transfusion of infected plasma or blood.

JAUNDICE—OBSTRUCTIVE

Condition. Obstruction to outflow of bile from liver.

Causes. Obstruction to common bile duct by gall-stones, carcinoma of head of pancreas, other tumours or enlarged lymph nodes, e.g. from carcinoma of stomach. Occasionally, obstruction within liver, in bile canaliculi ('cholestatic jaundice'), produced by drugs especially chlorpromazine.

Symptoms and Signs. Jaundice. Pale stools. Dark urine (bilirubin). Itching. Tendency to bleed. Bradycardia. Perhaps pain.

Treatment. Treat underlying cause. Vitamin K_1 if prothrombin time abnormal.

Special Tests. Liver function tests at first normal, later abnormal—see above.

LEUKAEMIA (ACUTE)

Condition. An acute blood disease with malignant proliferation of white cells—either polymorphs, lymphocytes or monocytes.

Cause. Unknown. Increased incidence after much exposure to radiation, e.g. X-rays.

Occurrence. At any age.

Symptoms and Signs. General weakness and malaise. Anaemia. Haemorrhage from various sites. Ulceration of gums and throat. Bone and joint pains. Sometimes fever, respiratory infections. Liver, spleen and lymph nodes may be enlarged.

Treatment. Symptomatic, including blood transfusions. Combination cytotoxic chemotherapy in special centre. Steroids.

Special Tests. Blood count: low haemoglobin and red cell and platelet counts: white cell count greatly increased with many immature 'blast' cells. (White count may be normal or low in early stages—'aleukaemic' or 'subleukaemic'.) Prolonged bleeding time. Bone marrow biopsy shows marked increase in 'blast' cells.

Other Points. Fatal disease lasting a few weeks or months: temporary remissions occasionally occur spontaneously and may be produced by chemotherapy, prolonging life for up to two years. Prognosis is improving.

LEUKAEMIA (CHRONIC)

Condition. A chronic blood disease with great increase in white cells—either myelocytes ('myeloid') or lymphocytes ('lymphatic').

Cause. Unknown.

Occurrence. Commonest in middle or later life.

Symptoms and Signs. Gradual onset. Anaemia. Weakness. Anorexia. Haemorrhage from various sites. Enlargement of spleen with discomfort (gross in myeloid), of lymph nodes (especially in lymphatic) and of liver. A variety of symptoms due to leukaemic infiltration of various organs, e.g. skin, brain.

Treatment. General and symptomatic measures, including

blood transfusions. Specific treatment (not needed in early benign phase): (1) cytotoxic drugs; busulphan ('Myleran') in myeloid; chlorambucil ('Leukeran') in lymphatic; sometimes 6-mercaptopurine (myeloid) or cyclophosphamide (lymphatic): (2) radiotherapy—e.g. spleen irradiation or radioactive phosphorus: (3) rarely steroids: (4) occasionally splenectomy. Regular blood counts needed to regulate treatment..

Special Tests. Blood count: white cells greatly increased, often 500,000 per c. mm or more; few 'blast' (immature) forms. Haemoglobin and red cell counts low. Platelet count raised in myeloid in early stage. Bone marrow biopsy. Chromosomes and alkaline phosphatase of white cells are abnormal in myeloid.

Other Points. Fatal disease in 1 to 10 years (usually 3 or 4): terminally often changes to acute leukaemia or aplastic anaemia. Lymphatic type liable to infections.

MALABSORPTION SYNDROME

Condition. Faulty absorption in the gut leading to conditions of deficiency.

Causes. Surgical removal or reconstruction of gut. Hypersensitivity to gluten in coeliac disease and idiopathic steatorrhoea. Tropical sprue—unknown cause. Pancreatic disease or obstructive jaundice (causing malabsorption of fats and fat soluble vitamins A, D, E, K). Disease of small intestine—Crohn's, amyloidosis, connective tissue disorders or tuberculosis. Some drugs, e.g. neomycin.

Symptoms and Signs. Weakness. Loss of weight. Abdominal distension or discomfort. Diarrhoea, often with pale, bulky, fatty stool ('steatorrhoea'). Anaemia. Vitamin deficiencies.

Decreased calcium absorption (tetany, rickets, osteomalacia, bone pain, fractures). Pigmentation. Oedema. Clubbing.

Treatment. Treat cause if known. Low fat, high protein diet. Vitamins, calcium and iron. Gluten-free diet in coeliac disease and idiopathic steatorrhoea (see Coeliac Disease).

Special Tests. Haemoglobin and blood film. Serum electrolytes including calcium and phosphorus. Serum iron and B_{12}. Fat content of stool. Flat glucose tolerance curve. Xylose and other absorption tests. Barium meal. X-ray bones. Biopsy small gut mucosa.

Other Points. Prognosis varies with cause, but condition can usually be greatly improved.

MALARIA

Condition. General disease causing rigors and fever with splenomegaly.

Cause. Protozoa of genus Plasmodium. Enter stomach of Anopheles mosquito in ingested blood: multiply and reach its salivary glands, and are injected when it bites man: multiply in liver, then in red cells which rupture causing fever, etc.

Occurrence Very widespread—especially hot climates. Over 200 million cases a year.

Incubation Period. 1 to 2 weeks (up to 6 weeks for quartan).

Symptoms and Signs. Paroxysms: rigor, then fever, then sweating. Severe headache. Muscle pains. Vomiting. Enlarged spleen. Anaemia. Sometimes herpes labialis, jaundice.

Benign tertian (Plasmodium vivax): mildest form but most prone to relapse: paroxysms every other day: may be mild symptoms for 2 to 3 days beforehand.

Quartan (P. malariae): paroxysms ever third day: sometimes oedema, albuminuria, haematuria.

Malignant tertian, or estivo-autumnal (P. falciparum): paroxysms irregular, even continuous: severe because of complications due to infected red cells blocking capillaries—cerebral (hemiplegia, convulsions, delirium), pulmonary (haemoptysis), intestinal (vomiting, pain, melaena), shock and hypotension.

Blackwater fever (usually with falciparum): massive haemolysis causing jaundice, anaemia, haemoglobinuria ('black water'), often acute renal failure: mortality 25 per cent.

Complications. Ruptured spleen. Relapse due to parasites remaining in liver. Cachexia if chronic. Secondary infection.

Treatment. Chloroquine. Primaquine. (Quinine and mepacrine little used now.) Maintain fluids and diet. Analgesics. Sometimes blood transfusions. Blackwater fever—perhaps steroids, and treat acute renal failure if occurs.

Prevention. Daily proguanil ('Paludrine'), weekly pyrimethamine ('Daraprim') or chloroquine, Mosquito-nets at night, long trousers and sleeves and insect repellents by day. Drain breeding swamps of mosquitoes, or spray with insecticides.

May Resemble. Pneumonia. Acute nephritis. Infective hepatitis or Weil's disease. Acute abdominal conditions (see under Cholecystitis). Malignant tertian may mimic many diseases.

Special Tests. Examine blood films for parasites in red cells. White count low. E.S.R. raised. Urine for protein, blood, haemoglobin, etc.

Other Point. Notifiable disease.

Prognosis. Mortality is low with treatment, except in blackwater and cerebral complications of falciparum.

MARASMUS

Condition. Infantile wasting or failure to thrive.

Causes. Chronic underfeeding or wrong feeding. Kwashiorkor, due to protein deficiency. (Chronic infections, pyloric stenosis and some metabolic defects cause similar picture.)

Occurrence. Infants.

Symptoms and Signs. Failure to gain weight, or loss of weight. Wrinkled skin. May be diarrhoea or vomiting. Hypothermia. Oedema. Prone to infections.

Treatment. Keep child warm and guard from infection. Feeds: check quantities, times and methods of giving. Often necessary to change food. Vitamin supplements (especially A, C, D). Intravenous therapy if necessary—occasionally whole blood.

MEASLES (MORBILLI)

Condition. Acute infectious disease with symptoms similar to a severe cold, later followed by rash.

Cause. Virus.

Occurrence. Common disease, especially in winter. Epidemics occur. Chiefly children.

Incubation Period. 7 to 14 days.

Symptoms and Signs. Like severe cold: conjunctivitis, sneezing, headache, fever, cough, photophobia. Koplik's spots (small white spots on mucous membrane of cheek). Rash on fourth day: starts behind ears and rapidly spreads: macular, blotchy type.

Complications. Bronchopneumonia which may lead to bronchiectasis. Otitis media. Corneal ulcer.

Treatment. General measures. Treat complications.

May Resemble. Rashes due to drugs, serum or food. Scarlet fever. Rubella.

Nursing Points. Isolation for two weeks. Keep eyes, mouth and nose clean. Dark room if marked photophobia.

Other Points. Immunity usually permanent. Mortality chiefly from pneumonia, mainly in children under five, and in undernourished. Other complications occasionally. Active immunization may be achieved by injection of live attenuated vaccine. Injection of immune serum may protect or modify attack if given on exposure (before symptoms appear). Notifiable disease.

MEDIASTINAL OBSTRUCTION, PRESSURE OR INVASION

Condition. Pressure on (or malignant invasion of) surrounding structure by any mass in the mediastinum.

Causes. Large lymph nodes: carcinoma of bronchus or breast, Hodgkin's disease or lymphosarcoma, leukaemia, other malignancies, tuberculosis, sarcoidosis. Primary tumours (including retrosternal goitre). Aortic aneurysm. Pericardial effusion. Hiatus hernia. Mediastinitis.

Symptoms and Signs. Brassy cough, dyspnoea, stridor, pulmonary collapse and haemoptysis (pressure on trachea or bronchi). Hoarseness (pressure on recurrent laryngeal nerve). Horner's syndrome—ptosis, small pupil and lack of sweating on affected side of face (pressure on cervical sympathetic nerves). Venous engorgement of head, neck and upper chest (and perhaps arms) with oedema and cyanosis (pressure on superior vena cava). Dysphagia (pressure on oesophagus). Pericarditis. Chest pain.

Special Tests. Chest X-ray and barium swallow; perhaps screening. Look for primary tumour or accessible lymph node.

Biopsy enlarged lymph node elsewhere. Laryngoscopy. Bronchoscopy. Occasionally thoracotomy. Mediastinoscopy.

Treatment. Remove benign tumour. Radiotherapy often produces temporary shrinking in malignant tumours or lymph nodes.

MENINGITIS

Condition. Inflammation of meningeal covering of brain and spinal cord. Signs of meningeal irritation are neck stiffness, and pain on extending knee with hip flexed (Kernig's sign).

Causes. Infection with virus, meningococcus, other pyogenic bacteria, syphilis or tuberculosis. Similar signs occur without meningitis in some fevers in children ('meningism'), and in irritation by blood in subarachnoid haemorrhage.

MENINGITIS (VIRAL)

Causes. Various viruses. Commonest, acute benign lymphocytic meningitis. Also with specific fevers (e.g. mumps) and poliomyelitis.

Occurrence. Now commonest form of meningitis. Mainly in young people.

Symptoms and Signs. Acute onset with meningeal irritation and fever. Occasionally squint.

Treatment. Rest and symptomatic treatment.

Special Tests. Lumbar puncture—raised pressure and protein with lymphocytes. Sometimes virus studies on C.S.F. and blood.

Other Point. Almost all recover completely.

MENINGITIS—MENINGOCOCCAL
(CEREBRO-SPINAL FEVER)

Cause. Meningococcus: droplet infection.

Occurrence. Especially in young people. Often epidemics in schools, barracks and overcrowding.

Incubation Period. A few days.

Symptoms and Signs. Rapid onset. Malaise. Vomiting. Fever, Rigors (convulsions in children). Headache. Photophobia. Meningeal irritation. Irritability and confusion, later coma. Sometimes petechial rash ('spotted fever').

Complications. Bronchopneumonia. Deafness. Occasionally blindness, squint, paralysis, mental impairment or other brain damage. Hydrocephalus. Haemorrhage into adrenals with shock, cyanosis and collapse.

Treatment. Sulphonamides. Penicillin intramuscularly or intrathecally. Analgesics for headache. Sedatives. Lumbar puncture until C.S.F. sterile. Treat complications.

Special Tests. Lumbar puncture: fluid is turbid with many polymorph white cells containing meningococci: pressure increased. Naso-pharyngeal swabs, in early stages and for carriers.

Nursing Points. Darkened room. Give adequate fluid intake. Keep changing position. Care of skin, mouth, nose and eyes. Nasal feeding if unconscious. Burn swabs with discharges.

Other Points. Mortality high if untreated: up to 10 per cent even with sulphonamides. May be fulminating, ordinary or chronic types. May be infectious nasal discharge at onset or in carriers. Carriers may be symptomless. Notifiable disease.

Staphylococci, streptococci, pneumococci and other bacteria sometimes cause meningitis ('acute pyogenic meningitis'), usually secondary to infection elsewhere, e.g. pneumonia, osteomyelitis or spread from mastoiditis. Symptoms and signs similar but no rash. Diagnosis from C.S.F. Treat with sulphonamides and penicillin, or antibiotic indicated by the C.S.F. culture.

MENINGITIS—SYPHILITIC

Cause. Tertiary syphilis.

Occurrence. Usually within 5 years of infection with inadequate or no treatment but is rare. Very rarely, acute form in secondary stage.

Symptoms and Signs. Headache. Mental deterioration. Fits. Paralyses of various cranial nerves or limbs. Areas of anaesthesia, pain or wasting. Urinary incontinence. Meningeal irritation in acute form. Argyll-Robertson pupil and other features of tertiary syphilis.

Treatment. That of tertiary syphilis. Special treatment of symptoms.

Special Tests. Blood: V.D.R.L. positive. Cerebrospinal fluid: V.D.R.L. positive, lymphocytes increased.

Other Points. Slowly progressive, but can be arrested by treatment.

MENINGITIS—TUBERCULOUS

Cause. Mycobacterium tuberculosis: secondary to tuberculosis elsewhere—lungs, joints, etc., or miliary tuberculosis.

Occurrence. Any age, especially childhood.

Symptoms and Signs. Gradual onset. Lassitude. Increasing headache. Vomiting. Irregular fever. Confusion, especially in adults. Meningeal irritation. May be convulsions and paralyses of various cranial nerves and limbs. Coma. Perhaps those of tuberculosis elsewhere in body.

Treatment. General measures. Systematic and often intrathecal isoniazid (I.N.H.) and streptomycin. Sometimes P.A.S., 'purified protein derivative' (P.P.D.), steroids. If comatose, treat as for coma.

Special Tests. Cerebrospinal fluid: pressure increased, lymphocytes increased, tubercle bacilli may be found, 'cobweb' clot may form on standing. Air encephalogram.

Other Points. Fatal if untreated: with early treatment majority recover, but in some, paralysis or other symptoms remain.

MIGRAINE

Condition. Acute attacks of headache, prostration, eye symptoms and vomiting often with preceding aura.

Cause. Associated with abnormal constriction and dilatation of arteries inside and outside skull (in response to stimuli—alcohol, emotion, etc.). Rarely, maldevelopment of artery (e.g. aneurysm).

Occurrence. Commonest in early adult life, in tense precise personality, and when tired. May be family history.

Symptoms and Signs. Flashing lights or other visual changes. Perhaps sensory or motor loss mimicking a 'stroke'. Later, severe throbbing headache—usually one-sided. Photophobia. Nausea and vomiting.

Treatment. Analgesics in mild attacks, ergotamine if severe and possibly long term to reduce frequency of attacks. Cyclizine reduces vomiting. May need mild tranquillizers.

Other Points. Attack may last a few minutes or several days. Symptoms may be mild. Attacks often diminish in middle age.

MITRAL VALVE DISEASE

Condition. Deformity of mitral valve of heart following endocarditis. Regurgitation (incompetence)—failure to close. Stenosis—narrowing of orifice.

Cause. Rheumatic fever or chorea.

Occurrence. Commoner in females.

Symptoms and Signs. Dyspnoea on exertion. Orthopnoea. Palpitations. Cold, cyanosed face and hands ('malar flush'). Cough. Haemoptysis. Enlarged heart. Abnormal sounds and heart murmurs on auscultation. Angina.

Complications. Atrial fibrillation. Heart failure. Pulmonary hypertension in stenosis. Subacute bacterial endocarditis. Recurrent bronchitis and pneumonia.

Treatment. Regulation of life within capacity of heart. Surgery. Treatment of complications.

Special Tests. X-ray of heart (particular chambers enlarged) and lungs. E.C.G. Cardiac catheterization and angiography.

Other Points. Mitral stenosis is commoner: incompetence often occurs with stenosis. Patient often well for many years. Once failure occurs, progress to disablement in 3 to 10 years if untreated. Valvotomy (for stenosis) produces improvement for several years, but stenosis often recurs. Valve replacement (for incompetence with or without stenosis) much more hazardous.

MUMPS

Condition. An infectious disease with enlargement of the parotid, and sometimes other salivary glands: testis, ovary and pancreas sometimes involved.

Cause. Virus.

Occurrence. Common disease. Epidemics. Children and young adults.

Incubation Period. 14 to 21 days.

Symptoms and Signs. General malaise. Painful swelling of parotid and perhaps other salivary glands. Pain on moving jaws. Stiffness of neck. Orchitis: testicular atrophy and occasionally sterility may follow. Oophoritis (less frequently). Sometimes pancreatitis (abdominal pain and vomiting). Rarely encephalitis.

Treatment. General measures. Warm applications.

Nursing Points. Isolation. Keep mouth clean. May have to be fed through tube. Suspensory bandage if orchitis occurs.

MYASTHENIA GRAVIS

Condition. Weakness and rapid fatigue of some muscles.

Cause. Unknown defect of neuromuscular transmission—perhaps sometimes due to enlarged thymus or thymic tumour.

Occurrence. Commoner in females. Usually starts in early adult life.

Symptoms and Signs. Ptosis. Sometimes diplopia, facial weakness, defects in speech, swallowing and breathing. Later, limb muscles may be involved. All symptoms worse after use of muscles, recovering somewhat with rest. Thymus gland usually enlarged.

Complications. Respiratory infections and failure.

Treatment. Rest as necessary. Neostigmine. Pyridostigmine. If these drugs cause sweating, salivation or bowel colic, give atropine. Perhaps remove thymus.

May Resemble. Hysteria. Disseminated Sclerosis.

Special Test. Injection of edrophonium ('Tensilon') produces dramatic improvement for few minutes.

Other Points. Infections, emotion, childbirth and some drugs may aggravate symptoms. Remissions and exacerbations common. Some recover completely, others deteriorate over months or years, and 30 per cent eventually die of the disease.

MYELOMATOSIS (MULTIPLE MYELOMA)

Condition. Widespread malignant growths of abnormal plasma cells in bone marrow—ribs, sternum, spine, skull, pelvis.

Occurrence. Usually after age of 40 years.

Symptoms and Signs. Bone pain. If spine involved, cord or nerve damage may produce paralysis, root pain or sensory loss. Those of anaemia. Sometimes tendency to bleed. Liable to infections.

Complications. Fractures on slight stress ('pathological fractures'). Renal damage. Amyloidosis.

Treatment. Melphalan and other cytotoxic drugs. Radiotherapy to local lesions. Possibly steroids. Symptomatic—transfusions if anaemic.

May Resemble. Metastatic carcinoma. Osteoporosis. Hyperparathyroidism.

Special Tests. Blood: raised E.S.R.; anaemia, usually normocytic (i.e. with normal-shaped cells); later decrease in white cells and platelets; serum proteins abnormal with a characteristic globulin; serum calcium usually raised. Bone marrow: abnormal plasma cells. Urine: abnormal proteins present, e.g. Bence-Jones protein. X-ray: 'punched-out' translucent areas and pathological fractures or general rarefaction.

Prognosis. Usually fatal in a few years.

MYOCARDIAL DEGENERATION

Condition. Degeneration of the musculature of the heart.

Causes. Ischaemic heart disease. Hypertension. Any prolonged strain on heart, e.g. valvular disease. Vitamin B deficiency ('beri-beri') or alcohol. Endomyocardial fibrosis (tropical). Connective tissue disorders. Myxoedema or thyrotoxicosis. Amyloidosis or other rare infiltrative diseases. Cause sometimes unknown.

Symptoms and Signs. Tiredness. Dyspnoea. Heart failure. Arrhythmias (atrial fibrillation, etc.). Sometimes angina, heart block, fainting.

Treatment. Treatment of cause if known, and of heart failure.

Special Tests. Chest X-ray. E.C.G. Sometimes cardiac catheterization and angiocardiography. Exclude particular causes.

Other Point. Diphtheria, rheumatic fever and many infections may produce acute myocarditis but leave no after-effects if recovery occurs.

MYXOEDEMA

Condition. Diminished thyroid activity.

Causes. Thyroid atrophy (probably auto-immune process), partial thyroidectomy or treatment with radioactive iodine. Rarely secondary to hypopituitarism.

Occurrence. Usually middle age, especially women.

Symptoms and Signs. Slow mentality and movements. Husky voice. Dry skin. Feel the cold. Hair falling out. Constipation. Bloated face. Oedema which feels solid. Gain in weight. Slow pulse. Slow relaxation of tendon jerks. Anaemia. Menorrhagia.

Complications. Pericardial effusion and heart failure. Psychosis. Hypothermia and coma.

Treatment. Thyroxine (small doses at first, especially in old people, to avoid heart failure—increase gradually). Tri-iodothyronine if in coma.

Special Tests. Radioactive iodine uptake by thyroid, basal metabolic rate and protein bound iodine all low. Serum cholesterol raised. Blood count. X-ray heart. E.C.G. (low voltage).

Other Points. Insidious onset. Good prognosis if treated early, but hypothermic coma is usually fatal. For congenital thyroid deficiency, see Cretinism.

NEPHRITIS
(GLOMERULONEPHRITIS)

Condition. Non-suppurative inflammation of kidneys. The Ellis classification into Type I or Type II has been replaced by a pathological classification into 'proliferative', 'membranous' and 'minimal change' nephritis, according to the microscopic changes seen on renal biopsy.

ACUTE NEPHRITIS

Causes. Usually a hypersensitivity to haemolytic streptococci. Occasionally in connective tissue disorders.

Occurrence. Usually children and adolescents. Usually some days or weeks after a sore throat, scarlet fever or other haemolytic streptococcal infection.

Symptoms and Signs. Abrupt onset. Malaise. Headache. Fever. Oedema, especially puffy face. Diminished urine, haematuria. Usually slightly raised blood pressure, sometimes with heart failure and dyspnoea, and rarely, papilloedema, vomiting and convulsions ('hypertensive encephalopathy').

Treatment. Bed rest. Warmth. Diet: restrict fluids, low protein, no added salt. Penicillin. If convulsions, barbiturates and reduce blood pressure.

Special Tests. Urine: diminished volume, red cells and protein present, casts, may be high specific gravity. Blood urea raised. Occasionally renal biopsy.

Other Points. Ninety per cent recover completely; acute signs disappear after several days though renal function recovers more slowly. Ten per cent either die in acute attack, or after some months with progressive disease, or develop chronic nephritis years later. After recovery, infected tonsils may be removed with penicillin cover.

NEPHROTIC SYNDROME

Condition. Heavy proteinuria, generalized oedema, hypoproteinaemia and raised serum cholesterol.

Cause. May occur during the course of glomerulonephritis, in diabetes mellitus, amyloid disease (e.g. in longstanding rheumatoid arthritis) and sometimes in connective tissue disorders.

Occurrence. At any age.

Symptoms and Signs. Insidious onset. Often none until proteinuria present for some months. Gross generalized oedema. Renal failure and hypertension after some years.

Complication. Infections.

Treatment. Restrict salt and fluid intake. High protein diet unless blood urea rises. Adequate general diet. Diuretics. Steroids sometimes effective, especially in children with 'minimal change' type. Treat any infections.

Special Tests. Blood: raised cholesterol, lowered protein, normal urea levels (later, changes of renal failure). Urine: protein present, few or no red cells. Renal biopsy.

Prognosis—A few recover, but most die of renal failure after 2 to 20 years.

CHRONIC NEPHRITIS

Condition. End result of glomerulonephritis.

Causes. Some are of unknown cause. Hypertension, chronic pyelonephritis or any chronic renal disease produces similar end result. Symptoms, signs and treatment are those of Renal Failure (chronic).

NEUROSIS

Condition and Causes. Mental or physical symptoms arising from conflict or tensions, often unconscious; usually unsatisfactory personal relationships. Some hereditary disposition.

Types.

1. *Anxiety*—tension, fear, palpitations, lightheadedness, headache, dyspnoea, anorexia, nausea, vomiting, diarrhoea, tingling, lump in the throat, etc. Insomnia (especially hard to get off to sleep). May be exacerbations, as 'panic reactions', lasting some minutes.

2. *Obsessional or compulsive*—inability to rid mind of particular thoughts, or to avoid doing senseless things or repetitive actions.

3. *Hysterical* (see Hysteria).

4. *Depressive* (see Depression).

Treatment. Usually as out-patient unless symptoms disabling. Psychotherapy (also 'group therapy'—discussion in groups of patients). Reassurance that the patient will not become insane since anxiety about the outcome is often superimposed. Sometimes tranquillizers or night-sedation.

Nursing Points. Reassuring, friendly relationship helpful, but firmness necessary especially with hysterics. Do not blame.

Other Points. Neurotic reactions account for a considerable proportion of ailments seen by general practitioners. They are exaggerations of normal reactions to stress. Different from 'psychoses' (schizophrenia, manic-depressive psychosis, etc.) in that only part of the personality is involved, and the view of reality is predominantly normal—no gross delusions. Neurotics often 'rise to the occasion' in an emergency, psychotics do not. Considerable improvement often occurs, although may be chronic or recurrent. Complete recovery may occur if the underlying personality is sound, especially in acute neuroses precipitated by sudden stress (e.g. examination).

OSTEOARTHRITIS

Condition. Progressive chronic degenerative changes in synovial joints.

Causes. Commonly occurs with advancing age, with 'wear and tear'; especially in weight-bearing joints (spine, hips, knees), also elbows and fingers. Can also follow joint injury due to trauma, infection or other forms of arthritis.

Symptoms and Signs. Aching pain in joints especially after use, severe in later stages. Swelling and deformity of joints: bony outgrowths in fingers form 'Heberden's nodes' (especially in women). Creaking joints. Limitation of movement. Glossy white skin over joints. Muscular wasting.

Treatment. Avoid obesity. Avoid strain to joint. Local heat, e.g. wax baths, and active exercises. Analgesics, e.g. aspirin, phenylbutazone. Spa treatment: hot baths. Surgical treatment, especially for hip. Occasionally, injections into joint. Supports if spine involved.

Special Test. X-ray joints.

Other Point. May progress to bedridden disablement over years.

PAGET'S DISEASE
(OSTEITIS DEFORMANS)

Condition. Bony deformity especially of skull, spine, pelvis, limbs (especially legs). Local areas of increased destruction and formation of bone.

Cause. Unknown.

Occurrence. Late middle and old age.

Symptoms and Signs. May be no symptoms (disease found on X-ray). Painful, tender areas of bone, warm on palpation. Headache. Skeletal deformities with large head, kyphosis and bowed bones.

Complications. Fractures on slight stress ('pathological fractures'). Deafness. Renal calculi. Osteogenic sarcoma.

Treatment. Symptomatic. Occasionally calcitonin.

Special Tests. X-ray shows coarse distortion of normal trabecular pattern, with areas of sclerosis and translucency. Raised alkaline phosphatase. Serum calcium and phosphorus normal unless immobilized.

Prognosis. Chronic disease—may remain localized or gradually spread.

PARKINSONISM

Condition. Degenerative changes in part of brain (basal ganglia).

Causes.
1. Degeneration of unknown cause ('paralysis agitans').
2. Arterial Degeneration.
3. Encephalitis Lethargica.

Occurrence. Usually middle age. May be earlier, especially in post-encephalitic.

Symptoms and Signs. May begin with dragging or tremor of one leg. Stiffness and rigidity of muscles with slow, limited movement. Coarse tremor disappearing on movement and sleeping, with pill-rolling movement of hands. Expressionless face. Shuffling gait with quick small steps. Monotonous voice. Excessive salivation. Post-encephalitics may have 'oculogyric crises' (eyes turned upwards for seconds or hours). Occasionally, mental deterioration in post-encephalitic. May be finally bedridden and helpless.

Treatment. Regular protected life. Encourage and keep active as long as possible. Rhythmic co-ordinated exercises. Belladonna. Various proprietary relaxant drugs, e.g. 'Artane', 'Lysivane', 'Disipal'. Sometimes brain surgery.

Other Points. Chronic disease, may be progressive over many years. The recently-introduced drug L-Dopa makes management easier.

PEDICULOSIS

Condition. Infestation of the skin by louse which sucks blood. Three varieties: head, body, pubic louse.

Occurrence. Common with dirt and neglect. May occur in troops in the field.

Distribution. 1. *Head.* Especially in children. Louse becomes attached to the hair and lays eggs ('nits') which hatch out.

Scratching is frequent, and a secondary impetiginous rash occurs with enlarged glands in the neck.

Treatment. Comb out louse and eggs. Wash hair with paraffin. Gamma benzene hexachloride. Cut hair in very severe cases.

Distribution. 2. *Body.* Especially in adults and elderly. Chiefly trunk, thighs, buttocks. Severe itching, scratching; secondary septic rash.

Treatment. Gamma benzene hexachloride. D.D.T. powder. Disinfect clothes.

Distribution. 3. *Pubis.* Mainly in adults. Itching. Bluish bite marks.

Treatment. Gamma benzene hexachloride. D.D.T. powder. Shave hair. Disinfect clothes.

Other Points. All forms may need anti-pruritics and also antibiotics if secondarily infected.

PEPTIC ULCER

Condition. Ulceration of wall of stomach (G.U.), oesophagus or duodenum (D.U.).

Causes. Uncertain. Hydrochloric acid in gastric secretion plays a part. Sometimes related to mental stress. Steroids, aspirin, phenylbutazone and some endocrine diseases can cause or exacerbate them. Giant gastric ulcers associated with under-nourishment in elderly.

Occurrence. Any age—mainly between 20 and 60. D.U. is commoner in men than women (especially during reproductive period) and in professional classes rather than labourers. Also associated with race, blood groups, certain substances in gastric juice, and other hereditary factors.

Symptoms and Signs. Epigastric pain before (sometimes after) food, or at night, may radiate to back; relieved by alkalis or food. Vomiting which may relieve pain. Sometimes flatulence, heartburn, acid regurgitation, water brash, constipation or irritable colon. Epigastric tenderness. All symptoms periodic—occur for a few weeks at a time, with weeks or months free from them in between. Acute exacerbation with severe pain may simulate perforation.

Complications. Weight loss. Anaemia (due to slow bleeding). Severe haemorrhage with haematemesis and malaena. Perforation with peritonitis. Pyloric stenosis or hour-glass stomach, with vomiting of large quantities, including food eaten one or more days before; also sometimes succussion splash, visible gastric peristalsis and signs of malabsorption. Rarely carcinoma of stomach, from gastric ulcer.

Treatment. Avoid drugs listed under causes.

Acute symptoms: frequent alkalis (e.g. magnesium trisilicate, aluminium hydroxide, 'Nulacin'), milk, bland diet, propantheline. If necessary, bed rest, milk drip.

Complications: iron for anaemia. Blood transfusion or surgery for haematemesis or melaena. Perforation—surgery, with gastric aspiration and intravenous drip. Pyloric stenosis—surgery, after repeated wash-outs of foul stomach contents, and intravenous electrolyte replacement.

Long Term: eating 'little and often', taking alkalis, avoiding fried or spicy foods, may prevent symptoms. Medical treatment will not heal a duodenal ulcer, but should help it to heal spontaneously. Gastric ulcer helped to heal by 'Biogastrone' and giving up smoking. Surgery (vagotomy and pyloroplasty or gastroenterostomy, or partial gastrectomy)—heals most: indicated for troublesome, recurrent symptoms or complications.

May Resemble. Nervous or other dyspepsia. Cholecystitis. Carcinoma of stomach or pancreas. Diseases of other abdominal organs. Perforation resembles other causes of 'acute abdomen' (see under Cholecystitis).

Special Tests. Barium meal. Haemoglobin. Faeces for occult blood. Sometimes: gastric secretion tests ('test meals')—acid may be increased; gastroscopy.

Nursing Points. Watch for complications, e.g. rising pulse and falling B.P. in haemorrhage (may appear before haematemesis). Gastric aspiration (including secretion tests)—make sure tube is in stomach (test with litmus) and does not become blocked (blow air down; move tube if flow stops). Fluid chart—record vomit and aspirated fluid.

Other Point. Occasionally occurs elsewhere in intestine, e.g. in a Meckel's diverticulum, due to abnormal development of gastric-type mucosa there.

PERICARDITIS

Condition. Inflammation of the pericardium.

Causes. Cardiac infarction (may occur at the time or weeks after an infarct or cardiac operation or chest injury). Rheumatic fever or chorea. Connective tissue disorders. Infections—especially viral or tuberculous, or spread from adjacent sepsis or septicaemia. Uraemia (renal failure). Myxoedema. Tumours. Cause may be unknown.

Symptoms and Signs. Three types: 1. Acute, with chest pain, fever, friction rub on auscultation. 2. Effusion (may develop from 1), with no pain or friction rub, but breathlessness on lying down ('orthopnoea'), restlessness, engorged neck veins, fast weak pulse, low B.P., soft heart sounds on auscultation, and sometimes heart failure (from pressure on heart—'tamponade'). 3. Chronic constrictive (constriction of heart by scarred pericardium from 1 or 2, especially tuberculosis), breathlessness on exertion, heart failure.

Treatment. Rest. Treat cause and symptoms (pain, heart failure, etc.). If tamponade, aspirate effusion. Surgery for 3.

Special Tests. X-ray chest—heart shadow increased in 2; often calcified pericardium in 3. E.C.G. Perhaps aspirate effusion for cytology and culture.

Nursing Points. Frequent pulse and B.P. if acute—watch for tamponade.

Other Points. A few die in acute attack; most recover fairly completely.

PERIPHERAL NEUROPATHY
(PERIPHERAL NEURITIS)

Condition. Inflammation or degeneration of peripheral nerves.

Causes. Dietary deficiencies, e.g. vitamin B_1 and B_{12} (subacute combined degeneration of cord). Chronic alcoholism. Diabetes mellitus. Infections, especially viral (also diphtheria, leprosy). Poisons, e.g. lead, mercury. Drugs, e.g. nitrofurantoin, sulphonamides, phenytoin, INH. Cancer, especially of bronchus. Many cases are of unknown cause.

Symptoms and Signs. Pain, tingling and numbness in limbs. Diminished or altered sensation. Muscular wasting and weakness, especially of extensors (foot-drop, wrist-drop). Diminished or absent reflexes (especially ankle and knee jerks).

Treatment. Rest. Analgesics. Remove cause if known (e.g. control diabetes carefully). Prevention of deformity by splints. Passive and later active exercises. Electrical treatment. Vitamin B if appropriate.

Special Test. Measure nerve-conduction times electrically.

Other Points. All the above types tend to give widespread involvement—both legs and/or arms, mainly distally. Considerable improvement or recovery often takes place, except in diabetes and cancer. Some other diseases usually involve one nerve at a time, e.g. pressure on nerve from prolapsed intervertebral disc ('slipped disc') or tumour or other cause; polyarteritis nodosa. A special cause of painful, pinkish hands and feet and hypotonia (floppiness) in children is 'pink disease' or acrodynia, probably due to mercury poisoning: misery, photophobia, excessive salivation, rashes and more severe skin changes occur in this.

PITUITARY DISORDERS

Produce many symptoms and signs, as pituitary gland secretes many hormones, some of which control activity of other endocrine glands (thyroid, adrenal cortex, testes, ovaries). Tumours may lead to overactivity or, by pressure, to decreased activity of gland, to headache, or to partial blindness or diplopia due to pressure on cranial nerves 2 to 6.

DECREASED SECRETION

Dwarfism in children, with delayed mental, physical and sexual development.

Simmonds' disease in adults: usually due to infarction following post-partum haemorrhage, (Sheehan's syndrome); also after ablation of pituitary, e.g. in treatment of carcinoma of breast. Irregular menstruation or amenorrhoea, loss of pubic and axillary hair, myxoedema, Addison's disease, hypoglycaemia, coma especially if infection present.

Diabetes insipidus may co-exist with Simmonds'. Thirst and polyuria without glycosuria.

INCREASED SECRETION

Cushing's syndrome—see p. 37.

Acromegaly (or Gigantism in children). Acromegaly causes arthralgia, paraesthesia of hands and feet (e.g. carpal tunnel syndrome), enlarged bones especially hands, feet and head, enlarged liver, coarse features with thick skin, husky voice, headache, visual field defects, hypertension, diabetes mellitus; later weakness and deformities.

Treatment. If due to tumour, irradiation or removal. Give respective hormones in deficiency states.

Special Tests. Skull X-ray may show enlargement of pituitary fossa due to tumour. Glucose tolerance test, insulin tolerance test, thyroid function tests, urinary steroids and other tests of endocrine function.

PLEURAL EFFUSION

Condition. A serous effusion present between the two layers of the pleura.

Causes. Adjacent infection, e.g. pneumonia, tuberculosis. Malignant tumours of lung or pleura. Pulmonary embolus.

Symptoms and Signs. May be preceded by pleurisy. Dyspnoea; perhaps cyanosis. Fever and sometimes cough (depending on cause). Displacement of heart and trachea. Dullness and diminished chest movements on affected side with breath sounds and vocal resonance both diminished on auscultation.

Treatment. Treat cause. Breathing exercises. Aspirate fluid if much is present and to relieve distress.

Special Tests. X-ray chest. Culture sputum. Aspirate fluid for examination. Pleural biopsy.

Other Points. Sequelae: 1. absorption—leaving pleura

normal, or with adhesions, or thickened; 2. suppuration ('empyema'); 3. death, if terminal.

'Hydrothorax'—fluid transudate in pleural cavity without pleural reaction: occurs in heart failure, nephritis and other causes of oedema.

PLEURISY—ACUTE ('DRY')

Condition. Inflammation of pleura without much effusion.

Causes. As for pleural effusion.

Symptoms and Signs. Chest pain, worse on deep breathing. Shallow respiration with less rib movement on affected side. Dyspnoea. Fever and cough (depending on cause). Friction 'rub' and diminished breath sounds on auscultation over affected site.

Treatment. Rest. Analgesics. Heat to site (beware burns). If severe, injection of anaesthetic around intercostal nerves. Treat cause.

Other Points. Sequelae: 1. complete recovery; 2. pleural adhesions or thickening; 3. pleural effusion or empyema.

PNEUMONIA

Condition. Acute inflammation of lungs.

Causes and Occurrence. Infection with bacteria, virus or other organisms. Pneumococci usually affect one or more whole lobes ('lobar'); others (e.g. streptococci, staphylococci) usually produce diffuse changes throughout lungs ('bronchopneumonia'). Factors predisposing to pneumonia include bronchial obstruction (tumour or foreign body), aspiration of vomit, etc., other infections or lung diseases (measles, influenza, bronchitis), exposure to cold, old age or infancy, and general debilitation (e.g. 'hypostatic' pneumonia due to failure to cough up secretions, very common terminal event in comatose or bedridden patients, also post-operatively).

Symptoms and Signs. Usually rapid onset with chills, pleural pain, rising fever, headache, cough with rusty, bloodstained or purulent sputum, dyspnoea. Rapid respiration and pulse. Convulsions in children. Signs of consolidation—dullness and diminished chest movement with bronchial breathing and crepitations on auscultation. In severe cases, delirium, cyanosis, abdominal distension, cardiovascular collapse.

Complications. Herpes of lips. Pleurisy or pleural effusion. Empyema. Abscesses of lungs (and elsewhere in staphylococcal pneumonia). Bronchiectasis. Heart failure. Rarely meningitis, pericarditis.

Treatment. Bed rest. Warmth. Antibiotics (penicillin unless organism resistant). Oxygen, especially if cyanosis or tachycardia. Treat pain as for pleurisy. Breathing exercises and postural drainage to expand all lobes and bring up secretions. Occasionally, bronchial aspiration, bronchoscopy or tracheostomy necessary. Treat complications, and any associated diseases such as asthma.

May Resemble. Any acute infection in early stages. Acute abdominal disease (see under Cholecystitis).

Special Tests. Culture sputum for organism and its sensitivities to drugs. X-ray chest. Blood—white cell count and E.S.R. raised.

Nursing Points. Constant care. Position of comfort—usually propped up. Frequent drinks. Keep mouth clean. Suction or tracheostomy care if required. Watch for complications.

Other Points. Antibiotics very effective and frequently prevent severe disease. Pneumococcal pneumonia before antibiotics had mortality 25 to 50 per cent; now 5 per cent. Before antibiotics recovery was by 'crisis' (sudden fall of temperature, pulse, respiration) or 'lysis' (gradual fall): rarely seen now.

PNEUMOTHORAX

Condition. Air in the pleural cavity.

Causes. 'Spontaneous'—air may come from surface of lung, due to pleural tear or ruptured bulla in emphysema, tuberculosis, or in young people with no apparent cause. 'Traumatic'—air comes from outside of lung in penetrating wounds including pleural aspiration.

Symptoms and Signs. Pain in chest. Dyspnoea may be severe and progressive. Collapse, if severe. Displacement of heart and trachea. Less rib movement, with hyper-resonance and diminished breath sounds on affected side.

Treatment. Mild cases—rest and observation only; air reabsorbed spontaneously in two weeks. Severe cases—oxygen, analgesics, release air by inserting catheter into pleura. If persistent or recurrent—surgical treatment, or possibly inject irritant substance into pleural cavity (very painful). Treat wounds or tuberculosis.

Special Tests. X-ray chest. Sputum for tubercle bacilli.

Nursing Points. If pleural catheter draining to under-water seal, keep water bottle always below level of chest, or water will enter chest.

Other Points. May be 'valvular', i.e. air entering on inspiration with no escape on expiration—'tension pneumothorax', condition rapidly worsens. May be broncho-pleural fistula—persistent pneumothorax (often pyo-pneumothorax), treat surgically. Spontaneous pneumothorax may be recurrent.

Hydro-pneumothorax, accompanied by effusion. Pyo-pneumothorax, accompanied by pus. 'Artificial pneumothorax' is induced by a special apparatus in the treatment of pulmonary tuberculosis—rarely used now.

POISONING (ACUTE)

A great variety of drugs is taken in deliberate or accidental overdosage. The general treatment for many is as given for aspirin below. Household, garden or industrial chemicals often require special treatment. Details for individual poisons can be obtained by day or night by telephoning certain toxicology centres. Prevent poisoning in hospital by observing regulations, and at home by keeping drugs out of reach of children, and giving only limited supplies to depressed patients. Three common forms described below.

ASPIRIN

Symptoms and Signs. Headache. Tinnitus. Vomiting. Overbreathing. Dehydration. Hypotension. Coma. Sometimes haematemesis and melaena. Urine—positive ferric chloride test and reduces Fehling's. (Picture resembles diabetic coma.)

Special Test. Blood salicylate level. Blood gases, electrolytes.

Treatment. Maintain airway. Stomach washout. Artificial ventilation if necessary. Intravenous therapy to correct electrolyte disturbance and to promote diuresis. Perhaps dialysis (haemodialysis on 'artificial kidney' or peritoneal dialysis). Save urine and stomach washings. Treat as for coma.

BARBITURATES

Symptoms and Signs. Drowsiness and confusion. Coma. Tendon and corneal reflexes depressed or absent. Respiration quiet (later depressed)—patient looks asleep. Circulatory collapse. Death.

Treatment. As for aspirin poisoning.

Special Test. Barbiturate level in blood.

CARBON MONOXIDE (e.g. in car exhaust fumes)

Symptoms and Signs. Cherry-pink colour. Headache. Coma. Respiratory collapse. Circulatory collapse. Death.

Special Test. Spectroscopy of blood.

Treatment. Continuous inhalation of oxygen with 5 per cent CO_2. Artificial respiration.

N.B. Not found in 'natural' domestic gas (e.g. North Sea gas)

POLIOMYELITIS (ACUTE)

Condition. An acute infection sometimes attacking the spinal cord (anterior horn cells).

Cause. One of three viruses.

Occurrence. Chiefly children and young adults. Epidemics occur, especially in late summer.

Incubation Period. 3 to 21 days (usually 7 to 14).

Symptoms and Signs. Malaise. Headache. Fever. Sore throat. Nausea. Muscular pains. Later, mild meningitis with stiff neck, irritability. If paralysis occurs, may be one or two muscles or limbs, or whole body. Occasionally cranial nerves involved ('bulbar paralysis'), paralysing coughing and swallowing. Urinary and faecal retention occasionally (later recover).

Complications. Aspiration pneumonia and respiratory failure from respiratory and bulbar paralysis. Deformities following limb paralysis.

Treatment. Complete bed rest in isolation (activity in pre-paralytic phase increases severity of paralysis). Reassurance and often sedatives. Passive movements, active when fever settles. Cabinet respirator ('iron lung') or tracheostomy and respirator, if respiratory failure. Later re-education of muscles and orthopaedic operations for deformities.

May Resemble. Cold or influenza in early stages. Meningitis.

Special Tests. Lumbar puncture: cells and sometimes protein increased. Nasal swab and faeces for virology.

Nursing Points. Strict isolation. Avoid all effort for patient. Turn two-hourly. Fracture boards on bed. Support limbs, prevent deformities (sand bags to prevent foot drop). Disinfect faeces and swabs containing discharges. Tube-feeding, pharyngeal suction, catheterization if necessary. Special care when on respirator.

Other Points. Paralysis of limbs is maximum at first, or within a week. Any recovery of power starts within a month, but may continue for 6 months. Up to 50 per cent recover completely, 5 to 10 per cent die.

Tonsillectomy and routine injections should be avoided as far as possible during epidemics. Contacts should avoid severe exercise. Vaccines provide good immunity—oral type (Salk) now commonest. Carriers may be symptomless. Notifiable disease. Used to be known as 'infantile paralysis', but is *not* limited to infants.

PSORIASIS

Condition. Red areas of skin covered with silvery-white scales.

Cause. Unknown. Hereditary factor. May be precipitated or made worse by worry.

Distribution. Chief areas: front of knees, backs of elbows, lumbar region, scalp. Other areas: hands, nails, any area of skin. Often symmetrical.

Complication. Various types of arthritis occasionally associated.

Treatment. Topical applications: tar or steroid-based. Dithranol (stains clothing). Ultra-violet light. Rarely cytotoxic drugs.

Other Points. Fairly common disease. Tends to recur from time to time during lifetime of patient. General health may be good.

PULMONARY EMBOLISM

Condition. Foreign matter, usually thrombus, carried to lung by pulmonary artery.

Causes. Deep vein thrombosis. Myocardial infarction. Atrial fibrillation. Occasionally air or fat (after injury) or amniotic fluid.

Symptoms and Signs. Sudden chest pain and dyspnoea, perhaps with shock and cyanosis. Signs of right-sided heart failure. May progress to pulmonary infarction with haemoptysis, pleural pain or effusions, fever and shock.

Complications. May be rapidly fatal. Repeated emboli may occur and may lead to pulmonary hypertension and cor pulmonale.

Treatment. Bed rest. Avoid sudden effort to prevent further emboli. Oxygen. Analgesics. Anticoagulants. Perhaps antibiotics.

May Resemble. Cardiac infarction. Pleurisy. Pneumonia. Pneumothorax. Acute abdominal condition (see under Cholecystitis).

Special Tests. Chest X-ray. E.C.G. Culture sputum. Look for source of embolus.

Other Point. Incidence reduced by early mobility after operations.

P.U.O.
(PYREXIA OF UNKNOWN ORIGIN)

Reason that cause is unknown may be that symptoms of disease are minimal or that patient is unable to give adequate history, e.g. children, foreigners. May be a malingerer producing fever artificially. Careful examination of patient and urine will often reveal cause. Commonly due to infection of chest, urine, throat or ears. Other causes are deep vein thrombosis, subacute bacterial endocarditis, abscesses in abdominal or pelvic cavities, perinephric abscess, tuberculosis, brucellosis, typhoid fever, drug allergies, connective tissue disorders, reticuloses (e.g. Hodgkin's) and various tumours. Repeated examination of patient advisable for appearance of enlarged lymph nodes, heart murmurs, chest signs, etc.

Treatment. According to cause but preferably not before definite diagnosis made, or picture may be distorted.

Special Tests. E.S.R. White blood cell count. Chest X-ray. Examine sputum, blood, urine and faeces for pathogenic bacteria (and for parasites in stools). Blood agglutination tests.

Nursing Points. Make comfortable. Ensure adequate fluid intake—at least 3 litres per day.

PURPURA

Condition. Extravasation of blood into skin causing a blotchy type of rash: small spots—'petechiae'; larger bruises—'ecchymoses'.

Causes. Either reduced platelets or fragile vessel wall (or rarely coagulation defect such as haemophilia).

Allergies, drugs, infections or connective tissue disorders may cause either type. Reduced platelets ('thrombocytopenic purpura') also occur from unknown cause ('idiopathic thrombocytopenic purpura', especially in children and young adults), or secondary to bone marrow infiltration (especially secondary carcinoma), or to leukaemia, or in aplastic anaemia. Fragile vessel walls ('non-thrombocytopenic purpura') also occur in old age, scurvy, Henoch-Schönlein purpura.

Symptoms and Signs. Petechial spots or blotchy rash occurring anywhere on skin or mucous membranes. May be associated with bleeding elsewhere—from gums (especially scurvy) or nose, into gut, kidney, optic fundi, etc. Henoch-Schönlein purpura is a type of allergy to bacteria, or occasionally food or drugs: occurs especially in children and young adults, with bleeding into gut with abdominal colic and melaena, and into joints with swelling and pain.

Treatment. If severe, rest and transfusion with whole blood. Snake venom or special dressings to stop bleeding. Steroids and splenectomy in iodiopathic thrombocytopenic purpura, and occasionally in other types. Antibiotics if due to infection. Steroids or anti-histamines in Henoch-Schönlein. Vitamin C in scurvy. Treat cause if known.

Special Tests. Blood count (especially platelets). Bleeding and clotting times.

PYELONEPHRITIS (ACUTE)

Condition. Infection of kidney and pelvis of kidney.

Causes. B. coli commonly. Other bacteria include Proteus, Klebsiella pneumoniae, staphylococci, Streptococcus faecalis. Common with obstruction to flow of urine. Bacteria usually ascend ureter (see Cystitis), but may occasionally be blood-borne.

Occurrence. Commoner in females (especially in pregnancy).

Symptoms and Signs. Malaise. Fever. Rigors. Vomiting. Pain and tenderness in loin and flanks. Frequent painful micturition. Cloudy urine. Haematuria.

Treatment. Bed rest. Adequate fluid intake. Potassium citrate to make urine alkaline. Sulphonamides or antibiotics for several weeks. Remove obstruction.

May Resemble. Appendicitis. Gynaecological conditions. Renal calculus. Other causes of 'acute abdomen' (see under Cholecystitis).

Special Tests. Urine: bacteria (culture, sensitivity of organism), white cells, protein. X-ray: intravenous pyelography (I.V.P.). Blood urea and electrolytes. Check urine repeatedly for recurrence.

Other Points. If fully treated can be cured with complete recovery of renal function. If unrecognized or inadequately treated may lead to chronic pyelonephritis: this often produces no symptoms and is only found at routine medical examinations or when hypertension or renal failure results.

PYLORIC STENOSIS (ADULT)

Condition. Narrowing of pyloric outlet of stomach, causing obstruction.

Causes. Scarring after ulcer, especially duodenal. Gastric carcinoma near pylorus.

Symptoms and Signs. History of ulcer. Nausea. Vomiting of large quantities of foul material, including food eaten one or more days before. Visible gastric peristalsis. Abdominal 'splashing' on shaking ('succussion splash') even some time after meal. May be dehydration, wasting and other signs of malabsorption.

Treatment. Fluid diet. If more severe, repeated gastric aspiration and intravenous replacement of electrolytes and other deficiencies, followed by surgery.

Special Tests. Barium meal—large full stomach, emptying slowly and usually with signs of ulcer or carcinoma. Blood for electrolytes and haemoglobin. Perhaps histamine test: high acid suggests duodenal ulcer, absent acid suggests carcinoma.

PYLORIC STENOSIS (INFANTILE)

Condition. Narrowing of pyloric outlet of stomach causing obstruction.

Cause. Spasm or hypertrophy of pyloric muscle tissue, perhaps congenital.

Occurrence. Infants, within first two months. (Especially in second or third week.) Much commoner in males, especially first-born.

Symptoms and Signs. 'Projectile' vomiting. Wasting and signs of malabsorption. Dehydration. Constipation. 'Tumour' felt and sometimes seen in region of pylorus. Visible gastric peristalsis.

Treatment. Ramstedt's operation (division of muscle) after gastric washouts and intravenous correction of dehydration, anaemia, and other deficiencies. In mild cases, small meals and antispasmodic drugs ('Eumydrin', 'Skopyl') may be tried.

Other Point. Results of operation good if not too long delayed.

RENAL FAILURE

Condition. Failure of adequate renal function. May be acute or chronic.

Causes. Acute: Acute nephritis. Acute pyelonephritis. Hypotension (from haemorrhage, burns, dehydration, cardiac infarction or heart failure, septicaemia). Severe haemolysis (see Anaemia—Haemolytic). Poisons. Sulphonamides given with inadequate fluid intake. Acute urinary obstruction (e.g. calculi). Eclampsia.

Chronic: chronic nephritis (see p. 92), including chronic pyelonephritis, hypertension, diabetes or renal tuberculosis. Chronic urinary obstruction (e.g. enlarged prostate, ureteric calculi). Poisons. Connective tissue disorders (especially P.A.N. and D.L.E.). Polycystic kidneys.

Symptoms and Signs. Cerebral: headache, malaise, weakness, restlessness, confusion or depression, twitching or convulsions, sighing respirations, coma. Gastro-intestinal: vomiting, dyspepsia, distension, hiccough, constipation or diarrhoea, haematemesis and melaena. Cardio-vascular: hypertension (can be both cause and result of renal failure), heart failure, oedema and effusions, pericarditis. Liable to infections. Itching. Urine: specific gravity tends to be 1.010—small volume and dark in acute; normal or large volume often pale, in chronic (until terminal stage).

Treatment. Treat cause if possible. Controlled fluid intake:

daily intake usually equal to volume of urine + 500 ml in acute; high in chronic. Electrolyte correction as required: oral or intravenous alkalis, oral resins to absorb potassium ('Resonium—A'). Diet: high carbohydrate, low protein, to delay rise in blood urea. Treat haemorrhage or hypertension. Perhaps blood transfusions for anaemia in chronic. Dialysis if necessary in acute (haemodialysis on artificial kidney, or peritoneal dialysis); in chronic, this is practicable only occasionally and in otherwise fit people, since will have to be repeated regularly for rest of life. Replacement of kidney (in chronic failure) now becoming widely used. When recovery from acute failure begins, diuresis occurs, requiring large intake of fluid, salt and potassium. Onset of diuresis cannot usually be hastened by diuretics, (which are dangerous), but may occasionally by intravenous mannitol.

Special Tests. Repeated examination of urine, for cause and progress. Blood urea high. Plasma electrolytes abnormal (potassium high). E.C.G. (changes with high potassium). Haemoglobin. Chest X-ray (heart failure or pneumonia complicating). In chronic, I.V.P., cystoscopy, renal biopsy to exclude a remediable cause.

Nursing Points. Extreme accuracy in keeping fluid charts and administering correct fluid is life-saving in acute renal failure.

Other Points. Acute renal failure often recoverable, if patient can be tided over. Chronic is ultimately fatal, though progress may be delayed.

Renal dialysis units are in use in major hospitals all over the world, but are inadequate to treat the large numbers of people dying of renal failure. Home dialysis units are being set up, which patients manage themselves under supervision from a renal dialysis unit. Transplant now offers best hope.

RHEUMATIC FEVER (ACUTE RHEUMATISM)

Condition. An acute disease characterized by flitting arthritis and often cardiac involvement.

Cause. Probably a hypersensitivity to haemolytic streptococcal infections: commonly a few weeks after a sore throat.

Occurrence. Children and adolescents. Temperate climates.

Symptoms and Signs. Malaise. Tiredness. Fever. Sweating. Pain and usually swelling flitting from one joint to another, especially large joints. Subcutaneous nodules. Erythematous rash with raised margins ('erythema marginatum'). Erythema nodosum. Carditis: tachycardia and soft heart sounds due to myocarditis; heart murmurs due to endocarditis; pericarditis; heart failure. Chorea. Abdominal pain. Epistaxis. Pleurisy and pneumonia.

Complications. Heart valve disease (especially mitral, less commonly aortic). Sub-acute bacterial endocarditis.

Treatment. Rest in bed until pulse and E.S.R. normal. Penicillin. Salicylates. Steroids sometimes. Digitalis if heart failure. Chorea: see Chorea—Sydenham's.

Special Tests. E.S.R. Raised white cell count. Anaemia. E.C.G. Anti-streptolysin titre.

May Resemble. Acute osteomyelitis. Septic arthritis. Acute rheumatoid arthritis. Sub-acute bacterial endocarditis.

Nursing Points. Wrap joints in wool. Cradle. Absolute rest. Tepid sponging if high fever. Care of mouth and skin. Gradual return to full activity.

Other Points. Acute illness usually lasts 6 weeks, perhaps longer. Mortality in acute stage low. Attack may be mild and unnoticed—sometimes passed off as 'growing pains'. Further attacks common (and liable to produce serious cardiac injury). After first attack give prolonged penicillin or sulphonamides. Heart lesions may be discovered many years later.

RHEUMATOID ARTHRITIS

Condition. Chronic inflammatory changes occurring mainly in small joints.

Cause. Uncertain. Probably auto-immune disorder.

Occurrence. Commoner in females and in temperate climates. Usually starts in middle life. Also in childhood as 'Still's disease'.

Symptoms and Signs. Usually gradual onset. Malaise. Fever. Loss of weight. Anaemia. Tenderness and swelling of joints—hands, feet, wrists, ankles, knees, cervical spine. Movements restricted. Muscular stiffness and aching, worse in mornings. Wasting. Joint deformities, especially ulnar deviation of hand and spindling of fingers. Subcutaneous nodules, especially in forearm. Enlargement of spleen and lymph nodes, especially in Still's disease. Retarded growth in Still's disease.

Complications. Amyloidosis, may cause nephrotic syndrome (see Nephritis—page 91) and chronic renal failure. Inflammation of eye. Dry eye and mouth in Sjögren's syndrome. Leucopenia, fever, large spleen, weight loss in Felty's syndrome. Fibrosis of lung, especially on exposure to dust. Pleurisy.

Treatment. In acute attack: bed rest. Bed cage. Analgesics and anti-inflammatory drugs (salicylates, phenylbutazone, indomethacin). Immobilize inflamed joints with splints until less inflamed, then gentle exercises. Local heat. Steroid injections into worst joints: avoid systemic steroids if possible because of long-term complications (see Cushing's Syndrome). Gold injections (may also have severe side-effects).

In chronic stage: splints to joints at night. Local heat and active exercises. Rehabilitation. Surgery for severe deformities. Drugs as for acute attack.

May Resemble. Other forms of arthritis, including gout.

Special Tests. X-ray changes in joints. Anaemia. Raised E.S.R. Rheumatoid factor in blood—Rose-Waaler, latex and

D.A.T. tests. Urine for protein.

Nursing Points. Keep comfortable. Avoid pressure on tender joints. Care of pressure areas.

Other Points. Remissions and relapses over many years. Condition may remain mild or progress slowly or quickly to gross crippling. Osteoarthritis affects damaged joints.

RICKETS

Condition. Softening of bones due to poor calcium absorption due to lack of vitamin D.

Causes. Deficiency of vitamin D in diet, and lack of sunlight (which synthesizes vitamin D in skin). Malabsorption or renal failure can produce similar picture.

Occurrence. Usually children between 4 months and 2 years. Commoner in premature babies.

Symptoms and Signs. Flabby muscles. Prominent abdomen. Sweating. Irritability. Delay in dentition (with faulty teeth) and walking. Frontal bosses on skull, delayed closure of fontanelles. Enlargement of ends of bones, especially at wrists. Nodules where ribs meet costal cartilage ('rickety rosary'). Pigeon-shaped chest. Knock-knees or bow legs, and other bony deformities. Tetany.

Complications. Greenstick fractures. Stunted growth. Chest infections and emphysema. Small pelvis leading to difficulties in childbirth in women.

Treatment. Vitamin D and calcium, and foods containing them—milk, butter, eggs, cod or halibut liver oil. Sunlight or ultra-violet light. Treat tetany or malabsorption if present.

Special Tests. X-ray bones. Serum alkaline phosphatase high; calcium and phosphate may be low.

Nursing Points. Care in lifting child to avoid fractures.

Other Points. Prevent by good diet and sunshine, and supplements (but not an excess) of fish liver oils in first few years. Becoming rare in this country. Deficiency of vitamin D or calcium in adults causes osteomalacia.

RINGWORM (TINEA)

Condition. A fungal infection of the skin.

Cause. Contact with infected man or animal or with clothing, baths, etc.

Occurrence. Common disease, especially in children.

Symptoms and Signs. Circular reddish or scaly patches, with broken off hairs if on scalp. May occur on feet producing 'Athlete's foot', with moist flaking skin (especially between toes), or under nails making them rough, opaque and brittle. Tinea of groin (tinea cruris) may lead to large area of itching and soreness in groin. Common in young men.

Treatment. Griseofulvin by mouth. Whitfield's or other ointments (after cutting hair if on scalp): also powders, e.g. 'Mycil' if in sweaty area such as 'Athlete's foot', and keep dry.

Special Tests. Examination of hairs and scrapings from skin under microscope for fungus. Scalp lesions may fluoresce green under 'Wood's lamp' (U.V. light).

Nursing Points. Contagious. Avoid contact. Change socks or clothing daily if feet or body affected. Avoid walking in bare feet if feet affected.

RUBELLA (GERMAN MEASLES)

Condition. Infectious disease with rash and enlarged lymph nodes.

Cause. Virus.

Occurrence. Common disease. Epidemics especially in children.

Incubation Period. 14 to 23 days.

Symptoms and Signs. Symptom of head cold, sore throat and fever may occur one day before rash. Pale pink spotty or blotchy rash starting on face and neck, spreading to body and limbs, and generally lasting 2 or 3 days. Enlarged tender lymph nodes especially behind ears and over occiput.

Treatment. Isolation. General measures.

May Resemble. Measles. Scarlet fever. Infectious mononucleosis.

Other Points. Almost always a mild disease with complete recovery. Second attacks rare. If develops in mother in first 3 months of pregnancy, infant may have congenital abnormalities; so avoid contact with case in this period, and give gamma globulin if contact does occur. Immunization widely available.

SARCOIDOSIS

Condition. Disease affecting many systems, with lesions resembling those of tuberculosis.

Cause. Unknown.

Occurrence. At any age. Commoner in young adults and in rural areas.

Symptoms and Signs. Initially often fever, erythema nodosum and swollen painful joints. Later, lassitude, loss of weight and any of the following. Enlarged painless lymph nodes—hilar nodes enlarged on chest X-ray. Lungs infiltrated, with fibrosis and dyspnoea. Various types of skin nodules or rashes. Decalcification of bones. Heart, kidney, liver, spleen, eyes, sometimes involved. Parotid swelling and facial palsy. Various neurological symptoms.

Treatment. Symptomatic. Steroids if serious lesions develop.

May Resemble. Tuberculosis. Hodgkin's disease. Beryllium poisoning.

Special Tests. Kweim test. X-ray chest and hands. Mantoux usually negative. Serum gamma globulin increased. Biopsy lymph node or skin lesion. Haemoglobin, white count and E.S.R.

Prognosis. Usually self-limiting disease, but may last a few years, and lung fibrosis may leave severe respiratory disability. Occasionally fatal if involves vital organs.

SCABIES

Condition. A parasitic disease of the skin.

Cause. Acarus. The female burrows into the skin and lays eggs which hatch out and cause further lesions.

Occurrence. Common disease. Spreads rapidly by contact, with lack of general cleanliness.

Distribution. Webs of fingers and toes. Wrists. Inner side of elbows. Body.

Symptoms and Signs. Rash. Multiple small sinuous 'burrows' in skin. Severe itching, more marked at night. Scratch marks.

Complications. Impetigo. Eczematous rash.

Treatment. Hot bath followed by application of benzyl benzoate or gamma benzene hexachloride. May need anti-pruritic drugs (e.g. crotamiton) or antibiotics if secondarily infected. Daily change of underwear and bed linen. Treat contacts.

Special Test. The acarus can be seen under microscope after being removed from burrow by needle.

Other Points. Popularly called 'the itch'.

SCARLET FEVER (SCARLATINA)

Condition. An acute infectious disease with general malaise and an erythematous rash.

Cause. Haemolytic streptococcus.

Occurrence. Common disease. Especially children.

Incubation Period. 2 to 5 days.

Symptoms and Signs. Headache. Vomiting. Sore throat. Fever. 'Strawberry' tongue. Tender, enlarged tonsils and lymph nodes in neck. Rash—2nd day: rapidly spreading general erythema with darker spots, maximal in flexure creases; lasts a few days, followed by desquamation (scaling or flaking of skin).

Complications. Acute nephritis (type 1). Otitis media. Sinusitis. Suppuration of glands. Rheumatic fever.

Treatment. Penicillin. Treat complications.

May Resemble. Tonsillitis. Measles. Rubella. Infectious mononucleosis.

Special Tests. Dick test for susceptibility. Schultz-Charlton test sometimes in diagnosis.

Nursing Points. Fresh air. Warmth. Watch for complications. Care of mouth and nose.

Other Points. Infection usually through respiratory tract. May be through a wound ('surgical scarlatina') or through post-partum genital tract ('puerperal scarlatina'). Infection spreads from droplet infection, discharges, or spread by attendants by hands, milk, etc. May be carriers, e.g. convalescent patient.

Disease has declined in severity in recent years. With penicillin complications now rare. Second attacks rare. Notifiable disease.

SCHIZOPHRENIA

Condition. A progressive disintegration of personality.

Cause. Unknown. Hereditary factor. Attack may be precipitated by stressful situation.

Symptoms and Signs. Shallow or inappropriate emotional responses (e g. apathy, senseless smiles or grimaces, indifference to real or imagined misfortune, callousness). Inattentiveness. Feeling of unreality. Failure to establish normal rapport in conversation. Delusions, including paranoia (persecution feelings) and idea that remarks and news-items relate to patient. Hallucinations (usually auditory, occasionally visual, smell, etc.). Use of invented words ('neologisms') or private code in speech and writing. Immobility and catatonia.

Treatment. Unsatisfactory—aim to arrest process and to prevent further attacks. Often requires repeated admission to psychiatric hospital. Chlorpromazine or tranquillizers. Psychotherapy. E.C.T. if depression associated.

Other Points. Chronic schizophrenia usually results in progressive deterioration without recovery, but sometimes partial recovery occurs (allowing return to normal or sheltered life) or even complete recovery. Extreme emotional stress (e.g. in war), pregnancy or toxic-infective illnesses may occasionally precipitate schizophrenia, sometimes of an acute type which often recovers.

SCHISTOSOMIASIS

(BILHARZIA)

Condition. Disease of the tropics due to infestation with trematodes-Schistosoma.

Occurrence. North, Central and South Africa, South America, West Indies and Far East. Occasionally seen in immigrants in temperate climate.

Symptoms and Signs. Affects liver, urinary tract and central nervous system. May have fever, abdominal pain, hepatosplenomegaly, haematuria, anaemia or neurological signs.

Special Tests. Identify eggs in urine or faeces. Blood count.

Treatment. Antimonials. Emetine, Lucanthone. Treat anaemia.

Other points. Intermediate host is freshwater snail. Efforts to eliminate it will reduce incidence of the disease.

SCURVY

Condition. A deficiency disease characterized by swelling and bleeding of the gums and haemorrhages.

Cause. Deficiency of vitamin C (ascorbic acid).

Occurrence. Infants: especially bottle fed. Adults: diet lacking fresh vegetables and fruit, especially old people.

Symptoms and Signs. Tiredness. Anorexia. Bleeding into skin (first around hair follicles, then as purpura), from mucous membranes, and under periosteum (painful limbs, may look paralysed); occasionally into gut (melaena), joints and elsewhere. Swollen, infected gums (unless edentulous), loose teeth. Rib 'rosary' similar to rickets. Anaemia. Wounds may not heal well.

Treatment. Ascorbic acid and food containing it (especially citrus fruits, blackcurrants, tomatoes). Cooking destroys ascorbic acid. Mouth hygiene. If subperiosteal haemorrhage—wrap limb in cotton wool, splint, cage.

Special Tests. Low vitamin C concentration in plasma, white blood cells, and urine. Vitamin C saturation test. X-ray long bones in infants.

Other points. Prevented in infants by routine orange juice. Infections or pregnancy increase vitamin C depletion. Used to be common on long sea voyages. May be associated with other deficiency conditions.

SEPTICAEMIA

Condition. Presence and growth of bacteria in the blood.

Causes. Various bacteria: from infection in wound, uterus after delivery, throat or elsewhere. May complicate various acute infections, e.g. pneumonia.

Symptoms and Signs. Fever: may be swinging or persistently high. Rapid and feeble pulse. Rigors. Sweating. Weakness. Wasting. Anaemia. Rashes and purpura. Joint pains. Sometimes delirium.

Complications. Abscesses in various organs. Thrombophlebitis. Pleurisy. Pericarditis, acute endocarditis. Adrenal failure.

Treatment. Special nursing care. Antibiotics or sulphonamides. Fluids freely, including intravenous drips. Drain septic focus.

Special Tests. Blood culture. Blood count (anaemia).

Other Points. Bacteraemia—transient presence, without growth, of bacteria in blood. Pyaemia—circulation in blood of infective emboli which lodge in various sites, e.g. lung, liver, brain, kidney or superficial tissues, to form an abscess.

SMALLPOX (VARIOLA)

Condition. A disease characterized by malaise and widespread pustular rash.

Cause. Virus.

Occurrence. Recent work by World Health Organization has almost eliminated the disease. Small pockets remain in Ethiopia.

Incubation Period. Usually 12 days.

Symptoms and Signs. Headache. Malaise. Fever. Influenza-like symptoms. May be prodromal erythematous rash. Rash: third day, macules changing to papules, vesicles and pustules; pitting follows; all come in one crop. More on face, head and limbs than trunk, rarely in axillae (in contrast to chicken-pox where lesions are mainly on trunk and come in several successive crops). Secondary temperature rise at pustular stage, perhaps with ulceration of throat and conjunctivitis. In very severe cases, pustules may coalesce ('confluent'), haemorrhage may occur into them and elsewhere, pneumonia and heart failure may develop.

Complications. Secondary infection of skin lesions. Scarring from pitting of pustules.

Treatment. Isolation. Bathe pustules with mild antiseptic and soothing lotions. Treat secondary infection (antibiotics) and complications. Antiviral drugs may become useful.

Special Tests. Serum agglutination tests. Examine vesicular fluid under microscope for virus products in cells. Culture virus.

May Resemble. Chicken-pox.

Other Points. Vaccinate as prophylaxis and on exposure to infection. Mortality varies according to severity of attack and whether protected by vaccination. Similar but milder disease may be due to minor strain of variola. Isolate patients and contacts in fever hospital. Quarantine period 18 days. Notify Medical Officer of Health when smallpox suspected. Patient must be attended only by those recently vaccinated. Vaccination usually protects if recent, otherwise modifies attack. Vaccination may be followed by appearance of vesicles (generalized vaccinia) or rarely by encephalitis: these complications more likely if eczema present when vaccinated.

Prophylactic infant vaccination has been withdrawn in Great Britain, as the incidence of serious complications exceeds by far the incidence of the disease. Vaccination is still essential for those travelling to endemic area.

SUBARACHNOID HAEMORRHAGE

Condition. Haemorrhage from a vessel on surface of brain.

Causes. Usually congenital aneurysm. Less often, weakness of vessel wall is due to other malformation or to atheroma. Occasionally, bleeding is secondary to head injury or cerebral haemorrhage.

Occurrence. Chiefly middle age, but may occur in the young and elderly.

Symptoms and Signs. Occipital headache, irritability and neck stiffness in leaking stage. When rupture occurs, sudden, severe pain like blow on back of head; often unconsciousness. Usually no paralysis.

Treatment. General nursing care as for cerebro-vascular accident. Surgery sometimes to tie off the aneurysm. Analgesics for headache.

Special Tests. Lumbar puncture: increased pressure of spinal fluid, fresh blood at time of haemorrhage, yellow fluid after a few days. Carotid or other arteriogram to look for source of bleeding.

Other Points. May be fatal. Tendency to recur.

SULPHONAMIDES

Nature. Group of drugs having an action against many organisms, but resistant strains are developing.

Administration. Orally. By injection if unable to swallow. Increase fluid intake to prevent crystals in urine.

Uses. Sulphadimidine—well absorbed: meningococcal meningitis, urinary infections or after bladder catheterization. Phthalylsulphathiazole—poorly absorbed: gastro-intestinal infections and to sterilize intestine pre-operatively. Others include sulphadiazine (good for meningitis because gets into C.S.F. well; but greater risk of crystalluria), sulphamethizole ('Urolucosil'—especially for urinary infections), sulphafurazole ('Gantrisin'). Sulphacetamide eye drops for local infections.

Toxic Effects. Malaise. Depression. Nausea. Diarrhoea. Hypoglycaemia. Fever. Rash. Skin sensitization to light. Haematuria and anuria if crystals form in urine. Blood disorders—purpura, haemolytic and aplastic anaemia, agranulocytosis. Peripheral neuropathy.

Other Points. First effective antibacterial drugs discovered 1935 ('M and B 693' was sulphapyridine). Problem of bacterial resistance overcome by combination with other drugs as in 'Septrin', 'Bactrim' (sulphamethoxazole/trimethoprim).

SYPHILIS

Condition. A venereal disease with widespread manifestations.

Cause. A spirochaete, Treponema pallidum. Almost always transmitted by sexual contact, but oral lesions infectious in secondary stage. (For Congenital syphilis, see p. 129.)

Signs and Symptoms. About 30% of contacts develop symptoms. Very few of those infected die of the disease. Divided into three stages, plus late neurological and aortic complications.

Primary (10 to 90 days after infection). Chancre—indolent hard sore at site of contact (usually genitals, may be finger, mouth, breast, anus, etc.). Regional lymph nodes enlarged. Sometimes fever, malaise, headache. Untreated heals in 3 to 8 weeks.

Secondary (Usually 6 to 8 weeks after chancre). Generalized coppery maculo-papular rash common. On mucous membranes of mouth, genitalia and anus—silvery erosions ('mucous patches' or 'snail-track ulcers'), groups of moist papules ('condylomata lata'). Headache, spirochaetes in C.S.F., but rarely neurological complications at this stage. Generalized lymph node enlargement, inflammation in eye, irregular bald patches. Goes on to latent stage; no symptoms or signs.

Tertiary (Usually 3 to 10 years after infection). Gummata (or gummas)—nodules, which in skin may form hard ulcers and later thin scars. Occur in any organ, especially skin (often face, neck, limbs) and bone (skull). Last for months if untreated. May resemble malignancy.

Neurosyphilis. A. *Meningovascular*—see Meningitis, Syphilitic. B. *General Paralysis of Insane* (G.P.I.: 10 to 15 years after infection). Cerebral atrophy, with slowly progressive dementia (sometimes 'delusions of grandeur'), epilepsy, tremor, ataxia, paralysis, incontinence, slurred speech. Transient cerebrovascular accidents ('congestive attacks'—last 1 or 2 weeks). Argyll-Robertson pupils (constricting with accommodation but not with light). Optic atrophy may cause blindness. Usually associated with aortitis. C. *Tabes Dorsalis* (About 10 years after infection). Degeneration of sensory nerve roots and posterior sensory columns of spinal cord. 'Lightning' and 'girdle' pains, through limbs and around trunk. Paraesthesia and loss of sensation. Painless destruction of joints (Charcot's joints—especially knee). Perforating ulcers on soles and elsewhere. Ataxia, difficulty in walking and co-ordination. Hypotonia (flabby muscles) and absent reflexes. Fractures. Sphincter disorders (retention or incontinence, of urine or faeces). Impotence. Eye disorders—double vision, optic atrophy, Argyll-Robertson pupils. Other cranial nerves involved, e.g. smell, taste, hearing. Painful 'crises'—gastric (pain and vomiting), laryngeal (cough, dyspnoea), rectal, vesical, etc. Often associated with G.P.I., meningo-vascular syphilis and aortitis, and sometimes with psychosis (e.g. paranoid schizophrenia) and gastric ulcer.

Aortitis. Inflammation of first part of aorta, often with dilatation, aneurysm, calcification, aortic incompetence, angina.

May Resemble. Almost any other disease, in its various stages.

Treatment. Penicillin (other antibiotics only if patient sensitive to penicillin). Herxheimer reaction—fever with acute flare-up of symptoms, sometimes dangerous—may occur when treatment begins, from toxins from killed spirochaetes: sometimes prevented by previous course of steroids. Occasionally iodides; fever therapy (malaria) for resistant neuro-syphilis rarely used. Treat complications.

Special Tests. Spirochaetes seen on dark-ground microscopy in material from primary or secondary lesions. Blood— Venereal Disease Research Laboratory test (V.D.R.L.), Reiter's Protein Complement Fixation (R.P.C.F.), Treponema Immobilization (T.P.I.), Fluorescent Treponemal Antibody test (F.T.A.). C.S.F.—V.D.R.L., R.P.C.F., protein (especially globulin) cells. X-ray chest (aorta), skull, bones. E.C.G. Biopsy accessible lesion.

Other Points. Primary and secondary lesions infectious: later stages (from 2 years after infection), usually not. Many patients present at tertiary or later stage, not having noticed previous stages.

Congenital. Syphilis may be transmitted to fetus by infected mother. Often causes abortion or stillbirth. If survives, develops rhinitis ('snuffles'), rhagades (scars radiating from mouth), Hutchinson's teeth (notched incisors of second dentition), interstitial keratitis (inflammation and blurring of cornea), bony deformities (collapsed bridge of nose, 'sabre tibia'), and all the features of secondary, tertiary and neuro-syphilis (G.P.I. may develop at age of 6 to 21).

TEMPERATURE MEASUREMENT

Clinical temperature measurement has traditionally been carried out in Great Britain using the Fahrenheit scale. Many hospital boards have already changed to the Centigrade scale and the practice will become general.

Fahrenheit		Centigrade
32°F.	Freezing point	0°C.
68°F.	Working temperature	20°C.
98.6°F.	Normal oral temperature	37°C.
100°F.		37.8°C.

A simple way to convert from one to the other is:

To convert degrees F. into degrees C. deduct 32, multiply by 5, and divide by 9.

To convert degrees C. into degrees F. multiply by 9, divide by 5, and add 32 to the result.

TETANUS (LOCKJAW)

Condition. Severe disease characterized by painful muscle spasms.

Cause. Clostridium tetani produces toxin which acts on motor nerve cells.

Occurrence. Organism can enter through any dirty cut or abrasion, especially contaminated by soil (which contains Clostridia), and thrives if necrotic tissue present.

Incubation Period. Varies from a few days to several weeks. The longer the incubation period the less severe is the disease likely to be.

Symptoms and Signs. Wound may be slight or even unknown. Usually starts with stiff jaw and proceeds to difficulty in swallowing and spasms of muscle of face (causing 'risus sardonicus'), neck and trunk. Any stimuli may precipitate spasm. Fever.

Complications. Cyanosis and arrested respiration. Pneumonia.

Treatment. Immunization with anti-tetanus serum (less likely to be effective if previously given, but if so then give in very large doses unless test dose reveals allergy—beware anaphylaxis). Wound toilet. Penicillin or other antibiotics to counteract wound infection and possible pneumonia. Sedation. Nurse in quiet room with as little disturbance as possible. If severe, give muscle relaxants, tracheostomy and positive pressure ventilation. Treat then as for unconscious patient—see under Coma. Remember paralysed patient is fully conscious. Tetanus does not confer immunity and patients who recover should be actively immunized—see Prevention.

Prevention. By surgical toilet (to remove dead tissue) to all wounds, and perhaps prophylactic antibiotics. Active immunization by tetanus toxoid (A.T.T.) to whole population and boost every 5 years or after any dirty wound or 6 weeks after A.T.S. given.

May Resemble. In early stage, trismus from sore throat or dental abscess. Hysteria.

Prognosis. Formerly about 50 per cent died, but with modern treatment about 20 per cent.

TETANY

Condition. Muscle spasm due to increased excitability of nerves, due to decreased ionized calcium in blood.

Causes. Hysterical hyper-ventilation. Excessive vomiting or excessive alkali ingestion. Hypo-parathyroidism (e.g. parathyroids removed inadvertently at thyroidectomy). Malabsorption. Rickets or osteomalacia.

Symptoms and Signs. Cramps in limbs, tingling in hands and feet. Carpopedal spasm: characteristic position of hands; if not present, may be elicited by inflating sphygmomanometer cuff around arm above systolic pressure for 4 minutes—Trousseau's sign. Chvostek's sign—tapping facial nerve in front of ear produces spasm of facial muscles. In children—laryngeal spasm with high pitched cry, convulsions.

Treatment. Intravenous calcium gluconate. If vomiting, saline infusion. If hyper-ventilation, calm patient down: re-breathing into bag; later repeat over-breathing to demonstrate cause and allay anxiety. Treatment of underlying cause (including vitamin D, except for first two causes).

Special Tests. Serum calcium, phosphate and other electrolytes. Tests for the possible causes.

THROMBOPHLEBITIS

Condition. Thrombosis of veins (superficial or deep), usually in legs or pelvis.

Causes. 1. Sluggish blood flow in veins, during bedrest, in heart failure, dehydration or debilitation, or after cardiac infarction. 2. Increased coagulability of blood, particularly 7 to

10 days after surgery or childbirth. 3. Trauma to veins, or surrounding infection.

Symptoms and Signs. If in leg (*especially calf*): tenderness, warmth, redness or cyanosis over vein; more marked if infective or in superficial veins. Increased circumference; oedema; tender, hard veins sometimes palpable; fever; positive Homan's sign (pain in calf when foot dorsiflexed); 'white leg' if associated arterial spasm. *If elsewhere:* usually no signs except perhaps fever.

Complications. Pulmonary embolism. Permanently swollen leg.

Treatment. If in superficial vein, give firm dressing, phenylbutazone and penicillin. If in deep vein, bed rest, keep affected part still, elevate swollen leg, anticoagulants. If frequent pulmonary emboli, ligate vein above thrombosis. Elastic stocking for persistent oedema.

Other Points. Avoid slow venous blood flow, by early postoperative ambulation and avoidance of pressure on leg veins (pillow behind knees is bad), and by encouraging leg movements in bed, especially in old people in heart failure. Strictly speaking, 'thrombophlebitis' means thrombosis with inflammation, 'phlebothrombosis' means thrombosis without inflammation. The greater the inflammation, the less the risk of embolism.

THYROTOXICOSIS
(HYPERTHYROIDISM, EXOPHTHALMIC GOITRE, GRAVES' DISEASE)

Condition. Enlargement of thyroid gland, with symptoms of general bodily disturbance and raised metabolic rate.

Cause. Excessive secretion of thyroid hormone.

Occurrence. Commoner in women, and before middle age.

Symptoms and Signs. Moderately enlarged thyroid, often with bruit heard over it. Tiredness. Nervousness and irritability. Tremor. Increased appetite with loss of weight. Prefer cold to hot weather. Sweating, warm skin. Palpitations. Rapid pulse (even when asleep). Prominent eyes (exophthalmos). Lid lag. Menstrual upsets.

Complications. Atrial fibrillation. Heart failure. Exophthalmos may cause paralysis of eye movements ('exophthalmic ophthalmoplegia') and damage to cornea. Muscle weakness (myopathy). Thyrotoxic crisis (rare now: usually precipitated by operation or infection, in untreated thyrotoxicosis)—delirium, diarrhoea and vomiting, heart failure, collapse—often fatal.

Treatment. Reduce thyroid activity by either 1. carbimazole ('Neo-Mercazole') or other anti-thyroid drugs (for at least one year); or 2. radioactive iodine (single dose); or 3. thyroidectomy (after preparation with carbimazole to reduce activity, followed by iodides (e.g. Lugol's iodine) to make glands less vascular). Sedation if necessary.

Complications of Treatment. Goitre often enlarges on carbimazole (very occasionally causing tracheal obstruction if goitre is retrosternal), and thyrotoxicosis may relapse when stopped. Occasional side-effects of carbimazole include agranulocytosis. Radioactive iodine may reduce activity too much or too little; it is not recommended in child-bearing years because of remote chance of ill effects from radiation. Thyroidectomy —too little or too much may be removed; recurrent laryngeal nerve may be injured causing hoarseness; parathyroids may be removed causing tetany. Exophthalmos may increase on any treatment.

May Resemble. Anxiety state. Other causes of weight loss, weakness, atrial fibrillation or heart failure.

Special Tests. Radioactive iodine uptake, protein-bound iodine (P.B.I.), raised. Thyroid scan may show 'hot nodule'.

Nursing Points. Weigh regularly. Special care before and after operation. Special care of eyes if exophthalmic.

TONSILLITIS

Condition. Inflammation of tonsils.

Cause. Usually haemolytic streptococcus.

Symptoms and Signs. Sore throat. Painful swallowing. Fever. Tonsils enlarged and red with yellowish white exudate which is easily removed. Lymph nodes enlarged in neck: perhaps a stiff neck.

Complications. Otitis media. Pharyngitis or bronchitis. Convulsions in children. 'Quinsy'—peritonsillar abscess. Rheumatic fever or chorea. Acute nephritis.

Treatment. Soothing gargles. Penicillin or other antibiotics.

May Resemble. Diphtheria. Thrush. Infectious mononucleosis.

Special Test. Throat swab.

Other Points. Recurrent attacks may lead to chronic infection. Surgery then indicated. In children, enlarged tonsils are frequently associated with enlarged adenoids causing mouth breathing, partial deafness and change in voice.

TUBERCULOSIS

Condition. Infectious disease involving lungs and many other organs, in which tubercles form (characteristic collections of cells and organisms, with caseation and later calcification).

Cause. Mycobacterium tuberculosis (human or bovine). Caught by droplet infection from man, or through infected cow's milk.

Occurrence. Commoner in pneumoconiosis, congenital heart disease, diabetes mellitus. Ill health, malnutrition and alcoholism lower general resistance and make widespread disease more likely.

General Characteristics. First (*primary*) infection with tuberculosis, usually in childhood, commonly occurs in lung, but may be in intestine, tonsil, skin or elsewhere. Regional lymph nodes enlarge and usually cause spontaneous cure by preventing further spread. Sometimes spread occurs, by lymph and blood, causing either 1. localized foci in other organs (kidney, bone, epididymis, etc.), which may heal or become latent, or 2. acute generalized 'miliary' tuberculosis or tuberculous meningitis (see under Meningitis), with death in few weeks if untreated.

A few weeks after primary infection, body develops hypersensitivity to tubercle bacilli (detectable by Mantoux test), and any subsequent (*post-primary*) infection—either from outside or by reactivation of latent focus—arouses much more local tissue reaction. This tends to confine the disease with less spread by lymphatics and blood, so less lymph node involvement and more local fibrosis and cavitation. Spread may occur through tubes—bronchi, oesophagus, etc. Runs a chronic course, until arrested by chemotherapy.

Symptoms and Signs. Primary. Often unnoticed. May cause fever for 1 or 2 weeks, erythema nodosum, and if in lung dry cough, pleurisy or pleural effusion. If in tonsil or intestine (infected by milk, rare now) usually no symptoms except enlargement of cervical or mesenteric lymph nodes. (Former may cause cold abscess behind angle of jaw. Latter, 'tabes mesenterica', occasionally causes abdominal pain, diarrhoea, malabsorption, ascites, intestinal obstruction.)

Acute miliary. (From blood-borne spread, usually in primary disease, sometimes from post-primary lesions anywhere in body.) Abrupt onset of fever, rigors, night sweats, prostration, headache, dyspnoea, sometimes signs of pneumonia or pleurisy. Lymph nodes, liver, spleen may be enlarged. Often tuberculous meningitis—see under Meningitis. If untreated, fatal in a few weeks.

Post-primary ('adult' type). Usually insidious onset, often no general symptoms. *Lung.* Productive cough, haemoptysis, altered sounds on auscultation (especially at apex), weight loss, malaise, night sweats. Sometimes pleurisy, effusion or abscess. *Intestine*, usually ileum. Sometimes diarrhoea, constipation, colic, appendicitis. *Kidney and bladder.* Urinary frequency and pain, haematuria, pyelonephritis, hydronephrosis, very small bladder. *Bones and joints* (especially spine—'Potts' disease'). Pain, swelling, destruction and sometimes ankylosis of joints. May discharge pus on to skin, or form cold abscess, e.g. in groin (tracks down psoas muscle from spine). *Skin.* Various lesions including reddish nodules on face and neck, with scarring ('lupus vulgaris'), or discharging sinuses or ulcers from underlying lymph nodes, usually cervical ('scrofuloderma'). Various rashes, including erythema nodosum, occur due to tuberculosis in other parts of the body.

Tuberculosis can also cause pericardial effusion leading to constrictive pericarditis, salpingitis leading to sterility, epididymitis, tuberculoma in brain, ulcer on larynx, pharynx or tongue (great pain on swallowing, hoarseness), inflammation in eye, and occasionally lesions in almost any organ of the body.

Treatment. Streptomycin, isoniazid (I.N.H.) and para-aminosalicylic acid (P.A.S.)—usually 2 or 3 together, to avoid resistance to one (other drugs, e.g. ethionamide, rifampicin if resistance does develop). Continue for at least 2 years. Perhaps steroids if acutely ill. Bed rest if acutely ill. Fresh air, good food (especially dairy products, meat, fruit and vegetables) and rest, e.g. in sanatorium, increase patient's resistance but are now less important than drugs. Isolation if infectious—especially with infected sputum. Special treatment of tuberculous meningitis—see under Meningitis, Tuberculous. Surgery to immobilize affected part—thoracoplasty to collapse lung, arthrodesis for joint—rarely necessary now, though sometimes for Potts' disease. Sometimes remove affected part of lung. Special treatment of complications.

Prevention. Maintain good hygiene, nutrition and general health. Test dairy herds for tuberculosis ('tuberculin-test') and pasteurize or boil milk. B.C.G. vaccination if Mantoux negative confers considerable protection. Mass miniature X-ray and checks on relatives of patients help early detection.

Special Tests. Examination of sputum, urine and discharges for 'acid-fast' bacteria (A.F.B.), and culture and guinea-pig inoculation (takes 6 weeks to grow). If no sputum—laryngeal swab, or bronchial or gastric washings. X-ray chest and other affected areas. Mantoux test (indicates only that infection has occurred—usually primary focus with complete healing, no longer active: but if positive to weak dilutions, e.g. 1: 10,000, often active). E.S.R., W.B.C. (often normal). Sometimes anaemia. Repeat sputum tests and X-rays for years to be sure relapse does not occur.

Nursing Points. Dispose of infected matter and articles. Maintain morale if long stay in hospital necessary.

Other Points. Majority of cases of tuberculosis can be completely healed (only tuberculous meningitis still carries considerable mortality), but if diagnosed late, serious damage may have occurred—destruction in lungs, short limb from joint involvement, destruction of kidney, small bladder. Some patients stop taking drugs—particularly P.A.S. which produces unpleasant indigestion: check on this, e.g. by testing urine for P.A.S. Pulmonary tuberculosis used to be called 'consumption' or 'phthisis'. Notifiable disease.

Incidence of tuberculosis diminished markedly after the introduction of anti-tuberculous chemotherapy. Incidence has remained at the same level for the last few years, but a higher proportion of notified cases now occurs in immigrants.

TUMOURS

Essentially tumours are new collections of cells which grow independently of normal body control mechanisms. These include abnormal tissue growths of all sorts. In behaviour they range from entirely benign ones (e.g. lipoma, fibroma) which do no harm except by pressure if near important structures and never recur if removed, through 'locally malignant' ones (e.g. rodent ulcer, parotid tumour) which invade surrounding tissue but do not metastasise, to highly malignant ones sending metastases by lymph and blood vessels to all parts of body, where new tumours form and eventually cause death. Carcinomas and sarcomas are all to some extent malignant.

Cure of malignant tumours is achieved if removed complete, before metastasising; or destroyed by radio-therapy (some tumours are sensitive to radiation, some not). Sometimes either method would cause too much damage to vital adjacent tissue.

Causes of tumour formation are generally unknown, but repeated trauma, irritant substances such as aniline dyes used in rubber industry (see Industrial Diseases, p. 67), excessive radiation or possibly viral infections can sometimes be responsible. Tumours may occur in any organ, and are dealt with in surgical books. The six below are selected because they are the commonest tumours and are commonly seen on medical wards.

BREAST—CARCINOMA

Occurrence. Commonest cause of female cancer death, particularly in middle-aged and elderly. Rare in men.

Symptoms and Signs. Lump in breast, often ignored for months by patient. Later, skin, nipple and axillary lymph nodes may become involved. Metastases commonly occur in bone, lung and liver.

Treatment. Simple mastectomy with or without radiotherapy. Radical mastectomy. Radiotherapy alone. Hormone therapy (oestrogen or androgen) useful in hormone dependent tumours. Oophorectomy, adrenalectomy, hypophysectomy may delay metastases. Cytotoxic drugs are sometimes used.

Special Tests. X-ray mammography, thermography in screening clinics.

Other Points. Prognosis good in earliest stage—women must be educated to inform doctor immediately of breast lumps.

CEREBRAL

Symptoms and Signs. Headache. Vomiting. Papilloedema. Failing vision. Slow pulse. Vertigo. Fits. Mental deterioration. Various types of paralyses and anaesthesia. Sometimes pituitary disorders.

Treatment. Surgical removal if possible. Relieve raised intracranial pressure by surgical decompression or hypertonic injections (urea or glucose intravenously, magnesium sulphate rectally). Treat epilepsy or other complications.

May Resemble. Other diseases of nervous system. Cerebrovascular lesions. Cerebral abscess. Uraemia. Psychiatric diseases.

Special Tests. Localization of tumour by detailed clinical examination, skull X-ray, angiography, air encephalogram. Lumbar puncture—pressure and protein may be raised: dangerous if intracranial pressure high.

Other Points. Cerebral tumour may be primary (e.g. meningioma, glioma), or secondary to growth elsewhere. Cerebellar tumours—prominent feature is staggering and falling to one side.

GASTRO-INTESTINAL—CARCINOMA OF STOMACH OR COLON

Occurrence. Middle and later life. Commoner in men.

Symptoms and Signs. Often none until late stage. Loss of weight. Anorexia. Nausea and vomiting.

Blood loss—gastric: haematemesis—colonic: rectal. Anaemia.

Pain—gastric: epigastric—colonic: colicky. Indigestion and flatulence. Obstruction—cardial: dysphagia—pyloric: persistent vomiting—colonic: 'acute abdomen'. Palpable tumour.

Signs of metastases: palpable in liver; jaundice due to bile-duct obstruction by lymph nodes; cervical lymph nodes hard (in gastric).

Treatment. Gastric. Gastrectomy seldom of lasting benefit. Palliative. Generally poor prognosis.

Colonic. Colectomy usually possible, colostomy otherwise. Prognosis quite good.

May Resemble. Gastric: peptic ulcer, pernicious anaemia. Colonic: diverticular disease.

Special Tests. Barium meal or enema. Occult blood in faeces. Gastroscopy. Sigmoidoscopy.

Other Points. Small bowel tumours very rare.

LIVER

Occurrence. Metastases common from carcinomas in alimentary tract. Primary tumours rare, commoner in negroes.

Symptoms and Signs. Large, hard liver, may be irregular. Ascites. General wasting. Occasionally jaundice, but rarely hepatic failure. Primary growth, outside liver, may produce other signs.

Treatment. Palliative. Sedatives. Tap ascites.

LUNG—CARCINOMA OF BRONCHUS

Occurrence. Commonest in middle life, and in males. Associated with cigarette smoking and certain industrial fumes. Commonest cause of cancer deaths.

Symptoms and Signs. May be none until late stage. Cough. Dyspnoea. Haemoptysis. Pain. Any of signs of mediastinal pressure or invasion, see under Mediastinal Obstruction. Pleural effusion, often bloodstained. Wasting. Superficial lymph nodes enlarged, hard.

Treatment. Surgical removal possible in a few cases. Radiotherapy may shrink tumour and reduce symptoms temporarily. Palliative. Sedatives. Oxygen. Tap effusion if dyspnoeic.

May Resemble. Chronic bronchitis, pneumonia, tuberculosis and other lung diseases.

Special Tests. X-ray (perhaps tomogram, bronchogram). Sputum or pleural fluid for malignant cells. Bronchoscopy. Mediastinoscopy. Biopsy tumour or lymph nodes. Exploratory thoracotomy may be necessary in some cases.

Other Points. Increasing in frequency. Multiple metastases often occur in lungs from cancer of other organs, e.g. breast.

TYPHOID AND PARATYPHOID FEVERS
(ENTERIC FEVERS)

Condition. An acute general infection causing ulceration of small intestine.

Causes. Salmonella typhi and paratyphi (A and B).

Occurrence. Less frequent with improvement in sanitation

and water supplies. Still occurs in tropics. Epidemics due to contamination of food or water, often by a 'carrier'.

Incubation Period. 1 to 3 weeks (usually 10 to 12 days).

Symptoms and Signs. 1st week: headache. Malaise. Rising remittent fever, but pulse rate not grossly raised. Epistaxis. Bronchitis. Constipation or diarrhoea. Furred tongue.

2nd week: rash from 7th day—rose spots on abdomen. Steady fever. Abdominal distension and discomfort. Soft, dark or 'pea-soup' stools. Spleen enlarged. Deafness. Sometimes muttering delirium. Pulse increased. Blood pressure decreased.

3rd week: unless complications or death occur, symptoms and fever lessen.

Complications. Haemorrhage from or perforation of intestinal ulcers in 2nd or 3rd weeks, or toxic myocardial degeneration—all grave. Pneumonia or thrombophlebitis early in convalescence. Relapse—usually mild. Late complications—bone abscesses, chronic infections of gall bladder or kidney.

Treatment. Maintain food and fluid intake, intravenously if necessary. Chloramphenicol, ampicillin. Treat complications, e.g. transfusion for haemorrhage.

May Resemble. Other diseases of intestinal tract. Pneumonia. Miliary tuberculosis.

Special Tests. Blood culture positive in first 2 weeks. White blood count low (high later, especially if perforation). Widal test, for salmonella agglutination, increasingly positive after 10 days. Stools and urine contain typhoid bacilli: test for patient being clear of infection in convalescence.

Nursing Points. Good nursing of paramount importance. General care of patient, mouth, skin, etc. Sponging if high fever. Disinfect soiled linen, stools and urine. Exclude flies. Boil crockery and feeding utensils. Scrupulous cleanliness of nurse and care of her hands. Encourage drinking ($2\frac{1}{2}$ litres a day) and taking of frequent small quantities of nourishing food. Watch for complications.

Other Points. Infection arises from food or drink contaminated with infected faeces or urine (water, milk, fresh vegetables, shellfish, etc.). Convalescent patient may remain as 'carrier' for a long time: bacilli in stools (from gall-bladder) or in urine (from kidney). 'Peyer's patches', lymphoid tissue in lower part of small intestine, are particularly affected. Paratyphoid infections usually milder than typhoid. T.A.B. inoculation gives considerable protection against enteric fevers for 2 years. Notifiable diseases. Other salmonellae can cause severe food poisoning.

TYPHUS

Condition. Group of related infections causing severe general illness and skin lesions. Includes 'epidemic typhus', 'scrub typhus', 'Rocky Mountain Spotted Fever', etc.

Causes. Various rickettsia: transmitted by lice (commonest type), ticks, mites and rat fleas.

Occurrence. Epidemics, especially during wars and famines.

Incubation Period. Usually about 12 days (can be 2 to 23 days according to type).

Symptoms and Signs. Usually abrupt onset with severe headache, generalized pains, rigors, flushed face with inflammation in eyes, nose, mouth. Bronchitis. Abdominal discomfort and constipation, with enlarged spleen. Fever rises for 3 days, lasts 2 weeks. Sometimes, deafness, photophobia. Rash: 5th day; rose spots, later dull, red-brown, not on face or palms. Nightmares, twitching, delirium and coma if severe.

Complications. Pneumonia. Otitis media. Parotitis. Renal failure. Gangrene and necrosis of skin. Myocarditis. Bleeding into skin, gut, urinary tract if very severe.

Treatment. Tetracycline. Chloramphenicol. Symptomatic.

Prophylaxis. Vaccines are available for most types. D.D.T. or other insecticides to remove lice, etc. Burn vegetation or otherwise disinfect or destroy wild or domestic animals on which fleas, mites and ticks live.

Special Tests. Weil-Felix (agglutination) reaction. Various other serological reactions and methods of culture.

Nursing Points. All attendants should wear protective clothing and insect repellents. Sterilize linen after soaking in disinfectant.

Other Points. Mild disease if actively immunized, when prognosis is excellent—without this or antibiotics 50 per cent may die. Even with recovery, mental power may remain impaired for 6 months or more. Those in contact with typhus, e.g. nurses, should be actively immunized. Has largely disappeared in areas with good housing and living conditions. Notifiable disease.

ULCERATIVE COLITIS

Condition. Chronic inflammation and ulceration of colon.

Cause. Uncertain. Food allergies and psychological factors may contribute. May be associated with auto-immune disease.

Occurrence. Especially young adults.

Symptoms and Signs. Attacks of diarrhoea with mucus and blood. Abdominal tenderness. Fever, anaemia and cachexia if severe.

Complications. Perforation. Pseudo-polyps. Stricture. Ischiorectal abscess or rectal fistulae. Carcinoma of colon. Generalized skin rashes. Arthritis.

Treatment. Replace water, electrolytes and blood. Sometimes milk-free diet. Diet rich in protein and vitamins (by gastric drip at night if nauseated). In acute attack, oral and rectal steroids, and perhaps sulphasalazine ('Salazopyrin'). (Rectal hydrocortisone can be given as a retention enema by the patient.) Perhaps antispasmodics (propantheline) and antibiotics. Iron between attacks. Treat complications. Surgical removal of colon (usually with ileostomy) if drugs ineffective.

May Resemble. Tuberculosis or cancer of bowel. Dysentery.

Special Tests. Examination and culture of stools (contain blood and pus). Sigmoidoscopy. Barium enema. Haemoglobin and plasma proteins (often low). E.S.R. (high).

Other Points. Attacks may be insidious or sudden, occasionally fatal. Usually runs chronic, intermittent course. May be signs of malabsorption. 4 per cent die in 1st year; 10 per cent in 5 years (was 30 per cent before steroids introduced).

URTICARIA (NETTLE-RASH)

Condition. Reddish-white wheals on skin (due to local oedema).

Causes. Allergy to foods (e.g. shellfish), drugs (e.g. penicillin, serum preparations), contact with animals or clothing. Infections, e.g. fungal or parasitic. Insect bites or stings. Physical factors, e.g. sunlight. Sometimes emotion plays a part. Cause may be unknown.

Symptoms and Signs. Perhaps malaise and slight fever. Severe itching of skin followed by erythema and wheals. Wheals come in crops and usually last a few hours but may be more chronic. Made worse by scratching. Occasionally blisters ('bullae') appear.

Treatment. Calamine or other lotions. Adrenaline if severe. Anti-histamines for treatment or prevention in susceptible people. Perhaps tranquillizers or even steroids. Avoid or treat cause if known.

Special Test. Skin test may show allergic cause.

Other Points. May be family history. In some people, urticaria can always be produced by firm stroking or 'writing' on skin ('dermographism'). 'Angio-neurotic oedema' or giant urticaria—larger swellings involving face (including eyelids), hands, genitalia; if mouth or larynx affected, can cause asphyxia.

VINCENT'S ANGINA

Condition. Ulceration of mouth and throat.

Cause. Uncertain. A spirochaete and a fusiform bacillus, both normal commensals, are found in large numbers.

Occurrence. Commoner in early adult life and in malnourished. Contagious especially amongst troops, in institutions, etc.

Symptoms and Signs. Sore gums and throat. Offensive breath. Red, bleeding gums. Painful greyish irregular ulcers in mouth and throat. Fever. Enlarged lymph nodes in neck.

Treatment. Dental care and oral hygiene—hydrogen peroxide mouth washes. Penicillin. Metronidazole ('Flagyl').

May Resemble. Diphtheria. Tonsillitis. Agranulocytosis. Acute leukaemia.

Special Test. Swab from mouth and throat.

Other Points. Separate utensils for patients. May become chronic. Also called 'ulcerative stomatitis'.

VITAMINS

Certain substances normally present in foods, the absence of which causes deficiency diseases. Only small amounts necessary.

A. Fat soluble. Present in fish liver oils, green vegetables, milk, eggs.

Deficiency causes xerophthalmia (thickening of cornea, etc.), night blindness, thick dry skin.

B. Water soluble. Many subdivisions:

B_1. Thiamin. Present in yeast, peas, beans, cereals. Deficiency causes 'beri-beri' (e.g. by eating polished rice)—heart failure and peripheral neuritis.

B_2. Riboflavin. Present in liver, eggs, milk. Deficiency causes stomatitis.

Niacin. (Nicotinic acid and nicotinamide). Present in meat, fish, cereals. Deficiency causes pellagra (dermatitis, diarrhoea, dementia).

B_6. Pyridoxine. Present in meat and vegetables. Deficiency causes stomatitis, peripheral neuropathy, convulsions.

B_{12}. Cyanocobalamin. Present in meat. Deficiency in diet or in absorption leads to megaloblastic anaemia (it is the extrinsic factor for the absorption of which 'intrinsic factor' absent from the stomach in pernicious anaemia, is necessary).

C. Water soluble. Ascorbic acid. Present in citrus fruits, blackcurrants, tomatoes. Deficiency causes scurvy.

D. Fat soluble. Present in fish liver oils, eggs, milk. Deficiency causes rickets, osteomalacia.

E. Fat soluble. Present in vegetable oils. Deficiency of doubtful significance.

K. Fat soluble. Exists as K_1 and K_2: latter unimportant so treat deficiency with vitamin K_1 or vitamin K analogue. Present in green vegetables. Deficiency causes bleeding tendency, through deficiency of prothrombin.

Other Points. Folic acid present in green vegetables and liver. Deficiency in diet causes megaloblastic anaemia, especially in pregnancy when requirements increase. Fat soluble vitamins not absorbed in obstructive jaundice.

WHOOPING COUGH (PERTUSSIS)

Condition. A respiratory tract infection causing a spasmodic cough.

Cause. Bordetella pertussis (Haemophilus pertussis).

Occurrence. Chiefly children under 5. Second attacks rare. May occur in the elderly.

Incubation Period. 7 to 14 days.

Symptoms and Signs. Starts like common cold. After 1 week, violent spasms of coughing producing thick sputum and followed by long-drawn inspiration (the 'whoop'). Cough may produce cyanosis and be followed by vomiting. Signs in chest of bronchitis. Sublingual ulcer may occur from friction of teeth on tongue protruded when coughing.

Complications. Bronchopneumonia, collapse of lung and later bronchiectasis. Occasionally coughing produces haemorrhage (purpura, epistaxis, even cerebral damage) or hernia.

Treatment. Fresh air. Tetracycline (only partially effective). Cough suppressant (e.g. linctus codeine) if severe. Treat complications, e.g. replace fluid, electrolytes and food if vomiting.

Special Tests. Incubate cultures of nasal swabs or special 'cough plates' that have been coughed on.

Nursing Points. Segregation in early stages only. Reassurance during spasms. Refeed if vomiting. Watch for complications.

Other Points. Vaccination (usually in form of 'triple vaccine' to cover diphtheria and tetanus also) gives some protection. Cough may take several weeks to disappear. Rarely fatal now —most deaths in infancy, due to pneumonia or cerebral haemorrhage or anoxia. Notifiable disease.

WORMS

HOOK WORMS

Two varieties—Ancylostoma and Necator—each about ½ inch long.

Transmission. Eggs passed in faeces: in soil soon become larvae which burrow through skin (especially bare feet): carried by blood stream to lungs: pass up respiratory tree and, being swallowed, change to adult form to become attached to wall of small gut and feed on blood.

Symptoms and Signs. None with mild infection. Sometimes skin reaction at site of entry with itching. Those of anaemia. May progress to heart failure. Epigastric discomfort, constipation (occasionally diarrhoea, vomiting).

Treatment. Tetrachloroethylene. Bephenium. Iron and well-balanced diet.

Special Tests. Ova in faeces. Anaemia—usually microcytic but later may be macrocytic. Eosinophilia. Occult blood in faeces.

Other Points. Only in those in or from warmer climates. With concurrent malnutrition, haemoglobin may reach extremely low levels, sometimes with comparatively few symptoms because of slow fall. Improve sanitation and wear shoes in endemic areas.

ROUNDWORMS (ASCARIS)

Appearance somewhat similar to earth worms—about 6 to 18 inches long.

Transmission. Eggs passed with faeces: become larvae in soil and thus transmitted by infected water or vegetables: once in small gut, migrate by lymphatics and veins to lungs and pass up respiratory tree to be swallowed: adult worms then live in small gut.

Symptoms and Signs. Abdominal pain. Cough and perhaps pneumonia or asthma when passing out of lungs. Urticaria. Worms may be passed or vomited or cause intestinal obstruction or perforation, or may migrate and cause abscesses, e.g. to liver, bile ducts, appendix, peritoneal cavity or up oesophagus to nose.

Treatment. Piperazine. Bephenium. Hexylresorcinol.

Special Test. Ova in faeces.

TAPEWORMS

Segmented worms of different types, may be several feet long. Head is attached to gut wall by suckers.

Transmission. Eggs passed in detached segments with faeces: become larvae in tissues when eaten by cattle, pigs or fish: infest man if such food is undercooked.

Symptoms and Signs. Often none. Passage of segments in faeces. Vague abdominal pains.

Treatment. Niclosamide. Dichlorophen. Mepacrine.

Special Tests. Segments or ova in faeces.

Other Points. Pig tapeworm larvae may invade subcutaneous tissue, muscle, brain forming cysts which may cause epilepsy, etc. ('cysticercosis'): above drugs may produce such invasion so treat pig tapeworm with male fern extract and bowel preparation. 'Hydatid cysts' in liver, lung, etc., due to larvae of another tapeworm—slowly grow and cause pressure symptoms, cough, haemoptysis, and if they rupture, allergic or toxic symptoms. Casoni skin test specific for hydatid disease: both types of cysts calcify and seen on X-ray. Treatment for both cysts is injection with formalin, or sometimes surgical excision. Fish tapeworm is a cause of megaloblastic anaemia.

THREADWORMS (OXYURIASIS OR ENTEROBIASIS)

About ½ inch long, like piece of cotton, living in caecum and surrounding gut.

Transmission. Eggs laid around anus especially at night and then carried to mouth or food on fingers or towels, etc.

Occurrence. Commoner in children.

Symptoms and Signs. Severe itching around anus. Worms in stool and around anus.

Treatment. Viprynium. Piperazine. Antipruritic cream to anus.

Special Test. Press 'Sellotape' to anus and examine microscopically for eggs.

Other Points. Treat whole household as others often unknowingly infected. Keep nails short. Wash hands after toilet and before preparing food.

YAWS

Condition. Non-venereal treponemal disease.

Cause. Treponema pertenue.

Occurrence. Primary infection ('mother yaw') usually occurs in childhood in areas of poor hygiene in the Caribbean, South America, Africa and Asia. There is a latent phase in adults. Complications may affect the bones, ear and eye uncommonly.

Special Tests. Serological tests for syphilis are positive.

Treatment. Penicillin injection (2.4 million units of long acting penicillin).

Other Points. Very common cause of positive serological tests for syphilis in immigrants from the endemic areas. Not transmitted to fetus.

INDEX

Abortus fever, 26
Addison's
  anaemia, 15
  disease, 9
Agranulocytosis, 9
Alcoholism, 10
Allergy, 11, 22, 54, 146
Anaemias, 11–15
Aneurysm, 16
Angina pectoris, 72
Angio-neurotic oedema, 147
Ankylosing spondylitis, 16
Anorexia nervosa, 17
Anthracosis, 69
Antibiotics, 17–20
Aortic disease, 20, 129
Argyll-Robertson pupil, 84, 128
Arterial degeneration, 21
Arthritis:
  osteo, 93
  rheumatoid, 116
Asthma, 22
Atrial fibrillation, 23, 86

Bence-Jones, test, 88
Beri-beri, 148
Bilharzia, 123
Botulism, 54
Breast, carcinoma of, 140
Bronchiectasis, 23
Bronchitis, 24
Bronchodilators, 22

Cancer:
  breast, 140
  gastro-intestinal, 141
  liver, 141
  lung, 142
Cerebral tumour, 140
Cerebrovascular accident, 27
Chancre, 128
Charcot's joints, 128
Chickenpox, 28
Cholecystitis, 28
Chloramphenicol, 18
Chorea:
  Huntington's, 30
  Sydenham's, 29, 115
Chvostek's sign, 132
Cirrhosis of liver, 30
Coeliac disease, 31
Colitis:
  mucous, 71
  ulcerative, 145
Collagen diseases, 33
Coma, 32
Connective tissue disorders, 33
Convulsions, infantile, 35
Coombs' test, 13, 60
Coronary thrombosis, 72
Cranial nerves, diseases, 35
Cretinism, 37
Crohn's disease, 17
Cushing's syndrome, 37, 65
Cystic disease of kidneys, 38
Cystic fibrosis, 39
Cystitis, 39

Depression, 40, 92
Dermographism, 147
Diabetes:
  insipidus, 100
  mellitus, 41

Dick test, 121
Diphtheria, 43
Disseminated sclerosis, 44
Duodenal ulcer, 96
Dysentry, 45

Eczema, 46
Emphysema, 47
Encephalitis lethargica, 48
Endocarditis, 49
Enuresis, 50
Enteric fever, 142
Epilepsy, 50–52
Erysipelas, 52
Erythema nodosum, 53
Erythroblastosis foetalis, 59

Farmer's lung, 68
Food poisoning, 54

Gastric:
  carcinoma, 141
  ulcer, 96
Gastritis, 55
Gastro-enteritis, infantile, 56
Gastro-intestinal cancer, 141
General paralysis of insane, 128
Glandular fever, 70
Goitre, 56, 133
Gonorrhoea, 57
Gout, 58
Graves' disease, 133
Gumma, 128

Haemolytic disease of new born, 59
Haemorrhagic disease of new born, 60
Hashimoto's thyroiditis, 11, 57
Heart:
  block, 61
  disease, congenital, 33
  failure, 62
  ischaemic disease, 72
  mitral disease, 86
  myocardial degeneration, 89
  myocardial infarction, 72
Heberden's nodes, 93
Henoch-Schönlein purpura, 110
Heparin, 72
Herpes Zoster, 28, 63
Herxheimer reaction, 129
Hodgkin's disease, 64, 81
Homan's sign, 133
Hookworm, 150
Hutchinson's teeth, 130
Hyperglycaemia, 42
Hypertension, 65
Hyperthyroidism, 133
Hypoglycaemia, 42
Hysteria, 66, 92

Icterus gravis, 59
Impetigo, 67
Industrial diseases, 67
Infectious mononucleosis, 70
Infective hepatitis, 74
Influenza, 70
Irritable colon, 71

Jacksonian epilepsy, 51
Jaundice, 73–75

Keratitis, 130
Kernig's sign, 82
Kwashiorkor, 80
Kweim test, 120

Lead poisoning, 68–69
Leukaemia, 12, 75–77, 81
Lice, 95

Liver, carcinoma, 141
Lockjaw, 130
Lung, carcinoma, 142
Lupus vulgaris, 137
Lymphadenoma, 64

Malabsorption syndrome, 77
Malaria, 78
Malta fever, 26
Mantoux test, 120, 136
Marasmus, 80
Measles, 80
   German, 33, 119
Meckel's diverticulum, 98
Mediastinal obstruction, 81
Meningism, 82
Meningitis, 82
Migraine, 85
Mitral disease, 86
Multiple sclerosis, 44
Mumps, 86
Myasthenia gravis, 87
Myelomatosis, 88
Myocardial degeneration, 89
Myxoedema, 89

Nephritis, 90
Neuritis, peripheral, 99
Neurosis, 92

Oesophageal web, 13
Ophthalmia neonatorum, 58
Osteitis, deformans, 94
Osteo-arthritis, 93

Paget's disease, 94
Parkinsonism, 48, 94
Paul-Bunnell test, 70
Pediculosis, 95
Pel-Ebstein syndrome, 64

Pellagra, 148
Penicillin, 18
Peptic ulcer, 96
Pericarditis, 98
Peripheral neuropathy, 99
Pertussis, 149
Petit mal, 52
Pink disease, 100
Pituitary disorders, 100
Pleural effusion, 101
Pleurisy, 102
Plummer-Vinson syndrome, 13
Pneumoconiosis, 69
Pneumonia, 102
Pneumothorax, 104
Poisoning, 105–106
   aspirin, 105
   barbiturate, 105
   carbon monoxide, 106
Poliomyelitis, 106
Postural drainage, 24
Pott's disease, 137
Prothrombin time, 73
Psoriasis, 107
Pulmonary embolism, 108
P.U.O., 109
Purpura, 110
Pyaemia, 124
Pyelonephritis, 111
Pyloric stenosis:
   adult, 111
   infantile, 112

Quinsy, 135

Ramstedt's operation, 112
Reiter's syndrome, 58
Renal failure, 113
Rhesus factor, 59

Rheumatic factor, 115
Rheumatoid arthritis, 116
Rickets, 117
Ringworm, 118
Roundworms, 150
R.P.C.F. Test, 129
Rubella, 33, 119

Sarcoidosis, 119
St. Vitus's dance, 30
Scabies, 120
Scarlet fever, 121
Schick test, 43
Schistosomiasis, 123
Schizophrenia, 122
Schultz-Charlton test, 121
Scrofuloderma, 137
Scurvy, 123
Septicaemia, 124
Shingles, 28, 63
Silicosis, 69
Simmonds' disease, 100
Sjögren's syndrome, 116
Smallpox, 125
Spastic colon, 71
Spectroscopy, 106
Still's disease, 116
Stokes-Adams syndrome, 20, 32, 62
Streptomycin, 19
Subarachnoid haemorrhage, 126
Sulphonamides, 127
Sycosis barbae, 67
Syphilis, 127–130

Tabes dorsalis, 128
   mesenterica, 137
Tapeworms, 151
Tetanus, 130
Tetany, 132

Tetracycline, 19
Threadworms, 152
Thrombocytopenic purpura, 110
Thrombophlebitis, 132
Thyrotoxicosis, 133
Tinea, 118
   cruris, 118
Tonsillitis, 135
Trigeminal neuralgia, 36
Trousseau's sign, 132
Tuberculosis, 136–139
Tumours, 139–142
Typhoid fever, 142
Typhus, 144

Ulcerative colitis, 17, 145
Undulant fever, 26
Urticaria, 146

Vaccination:
   BCG, 138
   smallpox, 125
Varicella, 28
Variola, 125
V.D.R.L. Test, 84, 129
Vincent's angina, 147
Vitamins, 147–148
   A, 148
   B, 14, 148
   C, 110, 123–124, 148
   D, 117, 132, 148
   E, 148
   K, 60, 148

Weil's disease, 74
Whooping cough, 149
Wood's lamp, 118
Worms, 150

Yaws, 152